24

Recent Advances in
Anaesthesia and Intensive Care

*Recent Advances in Ar   sive C   is the latest
book in this very succ   blis   titled
*Recent Advances in   y   n of
cutting-edge topics   the
world's leading au   ssful
formula of the prev   imes
have increased inr   larly
topical chapter o   aths
under anaesthesia,   ns   igeal
echocardiography   ainee   using an   and int   at all
levels will find thi book extremely relevant in   ir daily   ice.

Jeremy N. Cashman is a Consultant Anae   a   eorge's
Hospital, London and an Honorary Senior Le   An   ia at the
University of London.

R. Michael Grounds is a Consultan   aesthesia and Intensive Care
Medicine at St George's Hospital,   ion and an onorary Reader in
Intensive Care Medicine at the University of London.

24

Recent Advances in
Anaesthesia and Intensive Care

Edited by

Jeremy Cashman
Consultant Anaesthetist, St. George's Hospital, London
Honorary Senior Lecturer in Anaesthesia, University of London, UK

and

Michael Grounds
Consultant in Anaesthesia and Intensive Care Medicine, St. George's
Hospital, London
Honorary Reader in Intensive Care Medicine, University of London, UK

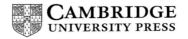

CAMBRIDGE
UNIVERSITY PRESS

CAMBRIDGE UNIVERSITY PRESS
Cambridge, New York, Melbourne, Madrid, Cape Town, Singapore, São Paulo

Cambridge University Press
The Edinburgh Building, Cambridge CB2 8RU, UK

Published in the United States of America by Cambridge University Press, New York

www.cambridge.org
Information on this title: www.cambridge.org/9780521706490

© Cambridge University Press 2007

First published 2007

Printed in the United Kingdom at the University Press, Cambridge

A catalogue record for this publication is available from the British Library

ISBN 978-0-521-70649-0 paperback

Every effort has been made in preparing this book to provide accurate
and up-to-date information that is in accord with accepted standards
and practice at the time of publication. Nevertheless, the authors,
editors and publisher can make no warranties that the information
contained herein is totally free from error, not least because clinical
standards are constantly changing through research and regulation.
The authors, editors and publisher therefore disclaim all liability for
direct or consequential damages resulting from the use of material
contained in this book. Readers are strongly advised to pay careful
attention to information provided by the manufacturer of any drugs
or equipment that they plan to use.

Contents

Contributors

Hannah Barrett
University Department of Anaesthesia & Intensive Care Medicine
N5 Queen Elizabeth Hospital
Edgbaston
Birmingham B15 2TH
UK

Julian F. Bion
University Department of Anaesthesia & Intensive Care Medicine
N5 Queen Elizabeth Hospital
Edgbaston
Birmingham B15 2TH
UK

Martin Bircher
Department of Orthopaedics and Trauma
St George's Hospital
Blackshaw Road
London SW17 0QT
UK

Alison D. Bullock
School of Education
University of Birmingham
Edgbaston
Birmingham B15 2TT
UK

Michael D. Christian
Mount Sinai Hospital and University Health Network
Toronto General

Toronto Western, and Princess Margaret Hospital
Room 18–206
600 University Avenue
Toronto M5G 1X5
Ontario
Canada

Brian H. Cuthbertson
Health Services Research Unit
Institute of Applied Health Sciences
Polwarth Building
Medical School
University of Aberdeen
Foresterhill
Aberdeen AB25 2ZD
Scotland

Peter Dieckmann
Danish Institute for Medical Simulation
Herlev Hospital
Herlev Ringrej 75
2730 Herlev
Denmark

Christopher Dodds
Professor, Cleveland School of Anaesthesia
James Cook University Hospital
Marton Road
Middlesborough TS4 3BW
UK

Lesley Durham
City Hospitals Sunderland NHS Foundation Trust
Royal Hospital
Kayll Road
Sunderland SR4 7TP
UK

S. Nicholas Fletcher
Department of Anaesthesia
St George's Hospital
Blackshaw Road
London SW17 0QT
UK

Anthony Gray
Department of Anaesthesia
Norfolk and Norwich University Hospital
Colney Lane
Norwich NR4 7UY
UK

Adrian Hall
Peter MacCallum Cancer Centre
East Melbourne VIC 8006
Australia

Stephen E. Lapinsky
Mount Sinai Hospital and University Health Network
Toronto General
Toronto Western, and Princess Margaret Hospital
Room 18–206
600 University Avenue
Toronto M5G 1X5
Ontario
Canada

Ian Loftus
Department of Vascular Surgery
The St George's Vascular Institute
St George's Hospital
Blackshaw Road
London SW17 0QT
UK

Scott Mercer
Pharmacy
St Thomas' Hospital
Lambeth Palace Road
London SEI 7EH
UK

Paul Older
Cardiopulmonary Exercise Testing Unit
Division of Anaesthesia and Intensive Care
Western Hospital
Melbourne VIC 3011
Australia

Rona Patey
Department of Anaesthesia
Aberdeen Royal Infirmary

Foresterhill
Aberdeen AB25 2ZN
Scotland

Marcus Rall
Universitatsklinikum Tuebingen
Abteilung fur Anaesthesiologie und Intensivmedizin
Tuebingen
Germany

Andrew Rhodes
St George's Hospital
Blackshaw Road
London SW17 0QT
UK

Kathleen M. Sherry
Ipswich Hospital NHS Trust
Heath Road
Ipswich
Suffolk IP4 5PD
UK

Thomas E. Stewart
Mount Sinai Hospital and University Health Network
Toronto General
Toronto Western, and Princess Margaret Hospital
Room 18–206
600 University Avenue
Toronto M5G 1X5
Ontario
Canada

Matt M. Thompson
Department of Vascular Surgery
The St George's Vascular Institute
St George's Hospital
Blackshaw Road
London SW17 0QT
UK

Shamim Umarji
Department of Orthopaedics and Trauma
St George's Hospital
Blackshaw Road
London SW17 0QT
UK

Preface

Every day you may make progress. Every step may be fruitful. Yet there will stretch out before you an ever-lengthening, ever-ascending, ever-improving path. You know you will never get to the end of the journey. But this, so far from discouraging, only adds to the joy and glory of the climb.
>   **Sir Winston Churchill** *British politician (1874–1965)*

As well as being the 24th edition of *Recent Advances in Anaesthesia* this will also be the 75th Anniversary edition. The series was first published as *Recent Advances in Anaesthesia and Analgesia (Including Oxygen Therapy)* in 1932. Since then there have been 23 editions. The title has been slightly changed over the years to reflect the changes in our practice, culminating in this the 24th edition of *Recent Advances in Anaesthesia and Intensive Care*. As in the past we have tried to ensure a range of topics encompassing basic science, clinical practice, new drugs and devices used in anaesthesia and intensive care, and in this edition the evaluation of training of the future generation of anaesthetists. We have chosen topics that we hope will be of interest to general anaesthetists as well as topics that may appeal more to the specialist anaesthetist and to the intensivist.

The first chapter by Drs Paul Older and Adrian Hall addresses a problem that many anaesthetists face: how to assess a patient with limited cardio-pulmonary physiological reserve who needs a major operation. Is it possible to determine in advance which patients are likely to present a major perioperative problem as a consequence of this limited reserve and how then to utilise our limited critical care resources for these patients. Surgery becomes annually more complex and many advances are driven by the fact that anaesthetists and intensivists are able to support the patients through this complex set of events. The next three chapters delve into different aspects of specialist surgery. In the second chapter, Dr Kathleen Sherry describes surgery and anaesthesia for oesophagectomy and considers the potential pitfalls. Professor Matt Thompson and Mr Ian Loftus, in Chapter 3, illustrate the advances in vascular surgery, an understanding of which will allow us to provide appropriate anaesthesia for the procedure being undertaken. In the last of this trio of chapters, Professor Christopher Dodds presents the difficulties that abound when faced with anaesthetising elderly patients with limited physiological reserve. Deaths solely caused by anaesthesia are very rare, but deaths where anaesthetic factors in combination with factors related to the patient's condition and to the surgery contribute to a patient's demise are more common. In Chapter 5, Dr Anthony Gray presents the lessons learnt from the UK National Confidential Enquiry into Perioperative Deaths (NCEPOD) regarding death caused by or following anaesthesia.

In the last few editions we have commissioned chapters on the care of patients under the broad heading of trauma, immediate care and resuscitation. Since 1998 there have been chapters on the Golden Hour, the Human Albumin Controversy, Resuscitation and Blunt Chest Trauma. In this edition we continue this trend with Chapter 6 by Shamim Umarji and Martin Bircher on the management of pelvic and acetabular fractures. Anaesthetists are inevitably involved in the care of these patients, either at the initial resuscitation stage or at the later reconstruction stage. The chapter gives good advice on our role in the care of these patients.

The next four chapters reflect advances in the world of intensive care medicine. Transoesophageal echocardiography (TOE) traditionally has been a tool used by cardiologists. However, recently many intensivists have begun to use TOE for intensive care patients. Chapter 7 by Dr Nicholas Fletcher describes the use of TOE by an intensivist rather than a cardiologist. Calcium sensitisers are a new class of positive inotropic drugs that are potentially useful in the treatment of acute decompensated heart failure. Levosimendan is the first intravenous calcium sensitizer to be approved in Europe for the treatment of acute decompensated heart failure. The drug is described in detail in Chapter 8 by Scott Mercer and Andrew Rhodes. There has been a significant drive over the past few years to provide 'intensive care without walls' and to extend some of the practices of intensive care to the general wards. Outreach has become 'de rigueur' throughout many healthcare services and is seen by many as the cheap alternative to intensive care units. Lesley Durham and Brian Cuthbertson review the case for and against outreach in Chapter 9. Critical care is often involved in the management of patients at times of biological disasters. The SARS (severe acute respiratory syndrome) outbreak was a good illustration of the need for critical care support. Michael Christian, Thomas Stewart and Stephen Lipinski review the role of critical care during such biological disasters in Chapter 10. Importantly they describe the lessons learned from SARS and the planning that is ongoing regarding any possible future pandemic.

Medical training is changing and this is particularly apparent in anaesthesia. The old system of apprentice-based training is gradually evolving into a more formalised (and very much shortened) training, with emphasis on ensuring that trainees are exposed to all aspects of anaesthesia. This being the case it is absolutely vital to ensure two things. Firstly, that all trainees are thoroughly assessed to ensure that they have reached an acceptable level of competency and knowledge before they finish their training. Secondly, that training programmes encompass all the aspects the trainees will need to be able to perform their tasks without supervision once they have completed their training. Hannah Barrett, Alison Bullock and Julian Bion describe in Chapter 11 how to assess a trainee's competence to leave the training grade. In Chapter 12, Dr Rona Patey focuses on how to develop processes that allow for lessons learned from previous events, to be incorporated into the training programme. It is the development of these behaviours to enhance safety and efficiency, which Dr Patey terms non-technical skills, that is an essential part of the new training process. The final chapter (Chapter 13) by Peter Dieckmann and Marcus Rall describes how the use of simulators can help with both assessments of training and of competency.

We are greatly indebted to all the authors who took time out from their already busy schedules to contribute to this latest edition of *Recent Advances in Anaesthesia and Critical Care*. We thank them for their enthusiasm and hard work. As with previous editions, *Recent Advances in Anaesthesia and Critical Care 24* aims to provide an up-to-date resumé on a wide variety of topics. We hope that the material presented herein has achieved that aim.

London
June 2007

J. N. C.
R. M. G.

Paul Older and Adrian Hall

The role of cardiopulmonary exercise testing in preoperative evaluation of surgical patients

The situation is, therefore, that the internist believes he can diagnose heart disease in life but can only state in a general way the patient's chance under operation; while the surgeon may deny this ability to discover heart disease while the patient is alive, but confidently makes such a diagnosis if the patient dies.

H. B. Sprague, 1929[1]

If this has a familiar ring then you should read on. Whilst this statement was made in 1929, the modern translation would still represent the feelings of many people today. One group would believe the first part and one group the second part. The true sceptic would of course believe both.

By virtue of the fact that the anaesthesia literature contains numerous articles discussing the best approach for preoperative assessment of major non-cardiac surgery with many urging caution and a rethink of the problem,[2,3,4,5] it is clear that the problem has not yet been solved! For example, some authors strongly recommend perioperative beta-blockade[6,7,8] and others are not so sure.[9,10] A recent systematic review, with meta-analyses, goes further and concludes that there is insufficient evidence to recommend perioperative beta-blockade in any type of surgery for the prevention of death, myocardial infarction or stroke.[11] How can there be such diversity of opinion with no resolution of such a common and serious problem? We believe that the reason for this is that too much attention has been focused on myocardial ischaemia as a risk factor. We also believe it is time to rethink the myocardial ischaemia paradigm which dominates most discussions on preoperative

Recent Advances in Anaesthesia and Intensive Care 24, ed. J. N. Cashman and R. M. Grounds. Published by Cambridge University Press. © Cambridge University Press 2007.

evaluation.[12,13] We hope that this article will offer a new perspective on these issues.

The current paradigm

The current paradigm for reduction of cardiac risk in non-cardiac surgery (preoperative testing for myocardial ischaemia and perioperative management including beta-blockade) targets only ischaemic heart disease. As explained by Kertai and colleagues,[14] plaque rupture accounts for only half of perioperative myocardial events, and prediction of perioperative myocardial infarction based on location and severity of coronary lesions is unreliable. We contend that perioperative cardiac morbidity in non-cardiac surgery has a different cause than cardiac morbidity in the non-operative setting. London and colleagues[8] suggest the myocardial oxygen supply–demand balance as another mechanism for major cardiac complications in non-cardiac surgery. The actual mechanism is unclear; they postulate a variety of aetiological factors, among which are impaired ventricular function and reduced coronary perfusion pressure. They acknowledge that 'limited physiologic data collection, most notably markers of the stress response or delineation of ventricular function have frustrated efforts to determine causal mechanisms'.

Non-cardiac surgery is a broad definition and encompasses procedures with large variations in postoperative stress response. Risk must be stratified according to patient-specific factors but also the surgery-specific risk,[15] i.e. the increased oxygen demand as a consequence of surgery. As London and colleagues imply,[8] the conventional paradigm ignores the important relationship between postoperative oxygen consumption and ventricular function. Preoperative evaluation must embrace more than just risk factor analysis for ischaemic heart disease; it should involve detection of all cardiac disease and, most importantly, objective assessment of functional capacity. The current obsession with one element of patient-specific risk, coronary artery disease, distracts attention from these other components of risk.

How do postoperative complications present?

The commonest presentation of postoperative cardiac complications is well known to most perioperative physicians; it is the patient who is hypotensive, tachycardic, oliguric and hypoxaemic in the ward two or three days following major surgery. This is often accepted as a manifestation of myocardial ischaemia progressing to perioperative myocardial infarction. However, these symptoms are equally those of a heart unable to meet the increased oxygen consumption of major surgery. We have already defined this syndrome as postoperative cardiac failure.[16] Under conditions of increased global oxygen demand following major surgery, it is probable that a heart with decreased functional reserve would exhibit signs of myocardial distress and damage. This would include sustained elevation of heart rate, arrhythmia, perhaps cardiac troponin release[14] and ECG evidence of ischaemia.[8]

Release of cardiac structural protein, i.e. troponins, does not necessarily imply myocardial infarction. Goto and colleagues[17] state that 'cardiac markers are quite sensitive to changes in left ventricular haemodynamic dysfunction', and that 'concentrations of the marker proteins appear to be related to left ventricular filling pressures'. Both of these conditions pertain to the postoperative period. Further, as Ammann and colleagues state,[18] 'the most important question is whether raised troponins reflect reversible or irreversible myocardial injury and how necrosis could be distinguished from reversible myocardial damage'. The end result of postoperative stress on a heart with decreased functional reserve may well be a progression to perioperative myocardial infarction, or to acute left ventricular dysfunction with overt pulmonary oedema or even to cardiac arrest. In these situations, as suggested by Sprague,[1] the diagnosis of ischaemic heart disease is made belatedly but with great confidence. However, as Kertai and colleagues[14] submit, correct postoperative diagnosis is frustrated by limited physiologic data collection.

A more frequent pathway of postoperative demise, as found in our studies[19,20] with monitoring of cardiopulmonary function and oxygen consumption postoperatively, i.e. with physiologic data collection, is dysfunction of other organ systems, a consequent requirement for haemodynamic support and a late progression to multiple organ failure. This is the sequence of primary postoperative cardiac failure, not primary myocardial ischaemia. The management of postoperative cardiac failure requires first a recognition that the morbidity is being caused by a failing heart which, in our view, would contraindicate beta-blockade; and secondly that treatment may require invasive monitoring and pharmacological support, which may include inotropes but rarely beta-blockade.

The diagnosis of postoperative cardiac failure should, of course, be made before progression to cardiac morbidity or to organ failure. Ideally, preoperative identification of patients at risk of this problem will result in modification of postoperative management, i.e. triage to monitored care in an intensive care unit, well before the patients at risk identify themselves by exhibiting the postoperative morbidity described above.

Cardiopulmonary exercise testing

We have shown that most perioperative cardiac morbidity in major non-cardiac surgery is related to cardiac failure, i.e. outcome is determined by the functional capacity of the cardiopulmonary system as determined by cardiopulmonary exercise testing (CPET).[19]

Performing the cardiopulmonary exercise test

Cardiopulmonary exercise testing involves computerised analysis of gas exchange and ECG data during exercise. The CPET is non-invasive. It consists of an exercise test with a progressive graded work rate and simultaneous breath-by-breath measurement, at the mouth, of inspired and expired concentration of oxygen and carbon dioxide, and inspiratory and expiratory gas flow. With this information oxygen uptake and carbon dioxide output may be derived. In addition a 12-lead electrocardiograph (ECG) is obtained continuously.

Our preference is to use a 'zero watt' cycle ergometer as the method of exercise. Compared to a treadmill, the cycle has the advantages of better isolation of lower limb musculature, less effect of movement artifact and greater safety because the subject is supported. Further, the workload can be varied in a step, incremental or ramp manner; these factors contribute to a more precise estimation of workload. A 'zero watt' cycle does not mean that the patient is performing no work, only that the patient is performing no 'extrinsic' work. The size of the patient, or more accurately the weight of the lower limbs, will dictate how much 'intrinsic' work is performed at 'zero' watts. The intrinsic work performed by the 'average' patient is approximately 25 watts. All the CPET at our laboratory were performed using a zero watt cycle ergometer (Corival, Lode®, Groningen, Netherlands) and a Cardi-O2 metabolic cart (MedGraphics Cardi-O2®, Medical Graphics Corporation, St Paul, MN, USA) and a computerised 12-lead ECG (Mortara ELI-100XR®, Mortara Instruments; Milwaukee, WI, USA). The manufacturers supplied upgraded software on a regular basis. The software of the metabolic cart was configured for continuous display of oxygen uptake, carbon dioxide output, work rate in watts, heart rate/VO_2 slope, ventilatory equivalents for oxygen and carbon dioxide (i.e. Ve/VO_2 and Ve/VCO_2), minute and tidal volumes and flow/volume loops and oxygen pulse (VO_2/HR), which is related to stroke volume.

The protocol for CPET was always the same. The metabolic cart was calibrated before each test and a medical specialist experienced in CPET supervised and reported all tests. Resuscitation equipment was available. A

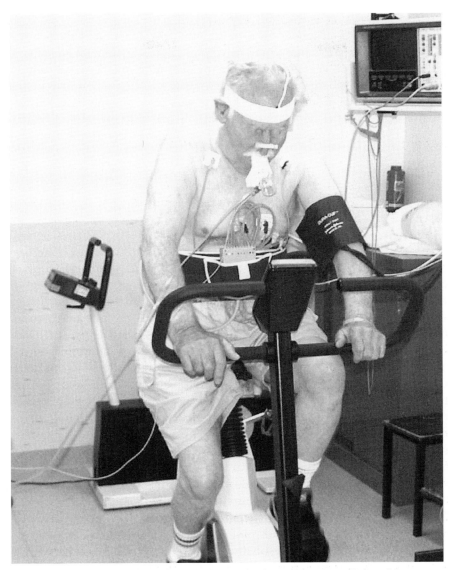

Fig. 1.1 A man on a bicycle ergometer during a CPET. Note the very small size of the mouthpiece and the extensive monitoring. (With patient permission: features altered digitally.)

12-lead ECG was obtained at rest and continuously during exercise and into the recovery period. The patient was seated on the cycle ergometer and the mouthpiece inserted (Fig. 1.1). Baseline gas exchange data were collected for approximately one minute. The patient then cycled against a zero watt extrinsic load for three minutes; for the next six minutes the extrinsic load was increased progressively using a ramp protocol to achieve the predicted maximum work rate. The algorithm for this was derived from Wasserman and colleagues.[21] It is of note that the duration of the test was slightly shorter than is often used in younger patients. Almost all patients tested were over 60 years of age and many over 80 years. We have found it difficult to motivate the elderly to cycle for much longer than nine minutes. All tests were symptom limited. The test was ceased if the ECG showed greater than 2 mm ST depression 60 ms after the J-point in any lead or if the patient became distressed. No effort was made to determine the peak aerobic capacity.

The primary determinant of cardiac function in our studies was the anaerobic threshold (AT). This was estimated using the 'V-slope' method described by Beaver and colleagues.[22] The anaerobic threshold is the point of oxygen uptake where anaerobic ATP (adenosine triphosphate) generation is needed to supplement aerobic metabolism. The anaerobic threshold has been used to define grading of cardiac failure.[23] Secondary criteria were determination of the nadir of the $V_E/\dot{V}O_2$ slope, the inflection point of the respiratory exchange ratio (RER), and the $\dot{V}O_2$ at which there was an increase in end-tidal oxygen concentration. All results were entered into a custom configured database that allowed calculation and graphical representation of derived data. The CPET is used to determine overall cardiopulmonary function and the precise cause of exercise limitation. As oxygen uptake is a function of ventricular performance, CPET may be used to define cardiac failure accurately without using 'estimates' or surrogates. As survival from major surgery is very dependent on cardiopulmonary function, as we will show later, CPET is used to accurately assess risk prior to major surgery. Much physiological data are accumulated during the test, which may be displayed graphically on a computer in 'real time' or stored for later analysis. This allows for comparison of two variables independent of time (bivariate analysis), which is the true power of CPET. There are 15 graphs, systematically arranged into nine panels: the 'nine panel plot' (Fig. 1.2). This plot is used to display the cardiovascular, ventilatory, ventilation/perfusion and metabolic responses to exercise. It is normally displayed in colour. For example, if oxygen uptake is plotted against work rate in watts, the slope of the line (or $\Delta\dot{V}O_2$/Work) gives a global assessment of exercise limitation. Similarly, carbon dioxide elimination plotted against oxygen uptake ($\dot{V}CO_2$ vs. $\dot{V}O_2$) is the basis for the 'V-Slope' method for determination of the anaerobic threshold. Ventilation/perfusion matching is evaluated by analysis of the relationship of oxygen uptake or carbon dioxide elimination to minute volume ($V_E/\dot{V}O_2$ or $V_E/\dot{V}CO_2$). The slope of the $HR/\dot{V}O_2$ plot is related to stroke volume and improves the accuracy of ECG diagnosis of myocardial ischaemia over ST segment analysis alone.[24] While these variables are not well known to most

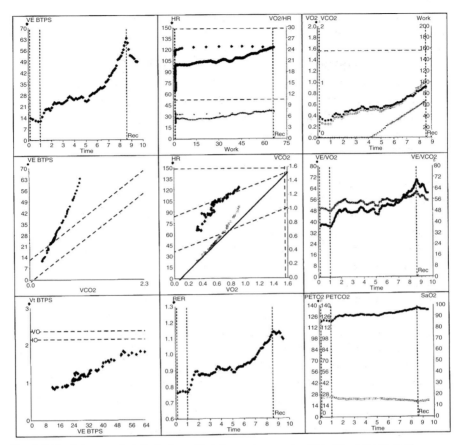

Fig. 1.2 The 'nine panel plot' displays 15 plots on nine graphs. This allows for ease of interpretation of the extensive data acquired from a CPET. It is normally in colour.

doctors, the normal responses to exercise are well defined; with appropriate display of data from CPET it is possible to determine the functional state of the entire cardiopulmonary system.

The risk factors

Cardiac failure not myocardial ischaemia

In a study of 548 consecutive elderly patients having major non-cardiac surgery and assessed by preoperative CPET, we examined outcome in relation to both cardiopulmonary function and myocardial ischaemia.[19] The incidence of myocardial ischaemia in these tests was 132 patients out of 548 (24%); most occurred as 'silent' ischaemia, i.e. without symptoms of chest pain. Of the nine deaths in the study attributable to cardiopulmonary causes, only one was caused directly by myocardial infarction. Only two deaths occurred in patients who had myocardial ischaemia, the other seven deaths occurred in patients with no evidence of ischaemia but with poor ventricular function. More importantly, there were no deaths related to cardiopulmonary causes in any patient with adequate ventricular function, defined as an anaerobic threshold above $11\,ml.kg^{-1}.min^{-1}$, even if myocardial ischaemia was present. If myocardial ischaemia were the dominant factor causing perioperative complications, such morbidity would occur predominantly in those patients with ischaemia. This is not the case in any of our published studies or unpublished series, now embracing over 1600 patients.

We conclude that it is the functional capacity of the heart and lungs, not the diagnosis of myocardial ischaemia, that determines the ability to support postoperative oxygen demand and thus influences morbidity and mortality after major surgery. Therefore, unlike the current paradigm for preoperative risk assessment, measurement of functional capacity and identification of cardiac failure is of prime importance.

Is myocardial ischaemia of no importance?

We do not intend to suggest that myocardial ischaemia is not significant. Myocardial ischaemia may well be a cause of poor functional capacity and thus, indirectly, perioperative death. However, we have shown that myocardial ischaemia is important only if it limits ventricular function.[25] Myocardial ischaemia in the presence of good functional capacity (defined as an AT greater than $11\,ml.kg^{-1}.min^{-1}$) was not associated with postoperative deaths in three published studies, one of 187 patients,[20] one of 214 patients, and one of 548 patients,[19] or a further unpublished series of 751 patients. The many studies that suggest myocardial ischaemia as the main cause of morbidity[26,6,7,27,28] did not evaluate ventricular function preoperatively in an objective fashion, if at all. Most studies make assumptions of the likelihood of myocardial ischaemia on a history of risk factors for coronary artery disease. When morbidity occurs it is attributed to coronary artery disease on the basis of these risk factors.

Risk factors for heart failure are often based on a history of hospital admission for acute left ventricular dysfunction. However, risk factors for cardiac disease in general, as well as for myocardial ischaemia, have the common end point of impaired ventricular function. It is our hypothesis that the patients who exhibit morbidity and mortality may well do so as a consequence of occult heart failure. This is by no means an uncommon problem.[29,30] Ignorance of heart failure as a major contributing factor to postoperative morbidity and mortality has other important consequences, not the least of which is that therapy is directed solely at prevention of myocardial ischaemia, including recommendations therefore for beta-blockade. A more logical approach would be to optimise cardiac performance and not just to concentrate on therapy for possible myocardial ischaemia.

Another perspective on myocardial ischaemia and cardiac failure

Our hypothesis emphasising the importance of heart failure in perioperative morbidity and mortality is supported by recent work from Hernandez and colleagues[31] in a series involving a study population of 3300 and a control group of 44 500. They showed that patients identified preoperatively with coronary artery disease (CAD) without heart failure, had a similar mortality to the general population (6.6% vs. 6.2%, $p = 0.518$, i.e. no significant difference) following major non-cardiac surgery. By way of contrast, those patients with heart failure had substantial morbidity and mortality (11.7% vs. 6.6%, $p < 0.001$). There were other significant findings related to readmission rates of the two groups. Heart-failure patients were readmitted more frequently for non-surgical reasons than the CAD group, with heart failure being the most common cause for this. Hernandez and colleagues[32] make the important point that 'the diagnosis of coronary disease was less important in heart failure patients because those with and without coronary disease had similarly poor outcomes'.

Assessment of functional capacity

The American College of Cardiology and the American Heart Association (ACC/AHA) Guidelines for Perioperative Cardiovascular Evaluation for Noncardiac Surgery[15] state, 'For patients with or without intermediate clinical risk factors, consideration of *functional capacity* (as determined by history of daily activities) and level of *surgery-specific risk* allows a rational approach to identifying which patients may most benefit from further non-invasive testing.' The guidelines also point out the reliability of functional status in prediction of cardiac events. They then state, '*If the patient has not had a recent exercise test*, [our italics] then functional capacity may be estimated from the ability to perform the activities of daily living.' Whilst this may be possible at the extremes of function it is not correct for the 'average' patient in the middle ranges of function, i.e. making a distinction between NYHA (New York Heart Association) class II and class III is extremely difficult, much more so than the distinction between class I and class IV. This was shown by Dunselman and colleagues in 1988 in a paper comparing CPET with clinical evaluation.[32] The conclusion of that study was that 'only data from exercise studies showed differences between the groups'. We consider that making a distinction between NYHA class II and class III is crucial for accurate preoperative assessment.

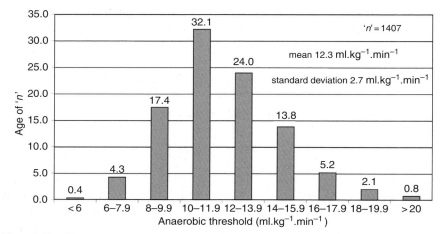

Fig. 1.3 The distribution curve of anaerobic threshold for 1407 surgical patients who underwent preoperative cardiopulmonary exercise testing.

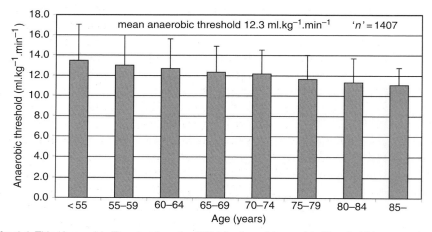

Fig. 1.4 Title 'Anaerobic Threshold vs. Age' Distribution of Anaerobic Threshold (mean and standard deviation) according to age group, for 1407 surgical patients who underwent preoperative cardiopulmonary exercise testing.

In all the studies that we have performed, the mean AT for patients over 60 years of age is 12.3 ± 2.7 ml.kg^{-1}.min^{-1} of oxygen uptake (Fig. 1.3). Using CPET data, Weber and Janicki[23] classified cardiac failure into five groups. In terms of AT, the range from no heart failure to significant heart failure is between 14 ml.kg^{-1}.min^{-1} to 8 ml.kg^{-1}.min^{-1}. In our series the mean, plus or minus one standard deviation, encompasses this range (Fig. 1.4). As our data show, patients at risk of perioperative cardiac morbidity have an AT of less than 11 ml.kg^{-1}.min^{-1} of oxygen uptake;[19] an AT of 11 ml.kg^{-1}.min^{-1} is within one standard deviation of the mean of our entire study population. Further, one standard deviation of any five-year age group of patients from 55 to 85 years of age embraces the mean of the entire cohort of patients. This clearly shows that age is not a valid discriminator of risk, a view supported by Wasserman.[33] Based on the above we do not believe it is possible to accurately identify all patients at risk of perioperative cardiac morbidity by age or by history and physical examination or to make a clinical distinction between patients with AT in the range from $10\,ml.kg^{-1}.min^{-1}$ to $15\,ml.kg^{-1}.min^{-1}$.

What is the best preoperative test of cardiopulmonary function?

With this in mind any preoperative test must be capable of defining cardiac failure at sub-clinical levels, as well as identifying myocardial ischaemia. In addition it should be non-invasive, objective and able to be performed at short notice on all patients, including outpatients. Time and cost are also important considerations. These desirable characteristics are the distinctive features of a cardiopulmonary exercise test. A CPET derives its information from measurements made on inspired and expired respiratory gases. A common criticism we face is how can a 'breathing test' accurately identify patients at risk of cardiopulmonary complications following major surgery? The answer is that CPET is not a 'breathing test'. The CPET involves accurate measurement of the physiological responses of the entire cardiopulmonary and circulatory systems under conditions of graded exercise stress. Whilst the physiology underpinning CPET has been appreciated since the time of Lavoisier in 1790[34] it did not become a clinically useful technique until nearly 200 years later. Incorporation into medical practice had to wait for the development of the technology to efficiently measure gas exchange on a breath-by-breath basis and to process very large amounts of data in real time. Currently, in CPET, cardiopulmonary data is displayed in graphical form. As various disease states show characteristic patterns of physiological response to exercise, interpretation of CPET is more easily achieved by examination of graphical data. This is far easier than interpretation of alpha-numeric data.

Estimates of functional capacity

Several studies[35,36,37] have shown that exercise capacity is a more powerful predictor of postoperative mortality than other risk factors for cardiovascular disease. It has also been shown that data from CPET predict long-term cardiovascular mortality in the general population.[38] The 2002 ACC/AHA Guidelines for Exercise Testing point out that the strongest and most consistent prognostic marker of poor prognosis is maximum exercise capacity.[39] The exercise capacity referred to here is only an estimate made in terms of metabolic equivalents (METs). A metabolic equivalent, or MET, is equal to the amount of oxygen consumed by a

40-year-old 70 kg male sitting at rest, and is equal to 3.5 ml.kg^{-1}.min^{-1} of oxygen uptake.

The Duke Activity Status Index (DASI) uses estimates of exercise capacity based on the energy costs of various activities, in terms of METs. A validation study of the DASI,[40] commented that 'DASI is an imperfect measure of exercise capacity. All three functional status measures tested in this study, including DASI, had poor correlations with measured exercise capacity in patients with peak oxygen uptake less than 5 METS. Thus DASI cannot replace exercise testing when a precise measurement of exercise capacity is needed. Bear in mind that 5 METs represent an oxygen uptake of 1225 ml.min^{-1} in the prototypical 40-year-old 70 kg male. This would relate, in our study population, to an AT of about 15 ml.kg^{-1}.min^{-1}, a figure achieved by less than 20% of our patients (see Fig. 1.2). In other words DASI, or other estimates, are not of value in the precise areas that surgical risk is increased. Many other commonly performed tests, as discussed later, including non-invasive exercise ECG,[41,42] radionuclide ventriculography,[43,33] echocardiography,[4] dobutamine stress echocardiography[5] and dipyridamole–thallium scintigraphy[2] do not evaluate functional capacity and have been proven to be inadequate for preoperative screening.[16] We feel that 'estimation' leads to unacceptable inaccuracy, particularly when functional capacity can now be measured accurately without difficulty.

Doing away with estimates and surrogates
The most reliable and objective test for measurement of exercise capacity is the CPET. Given that the role of the cardiopulmonary system is to enable gas exchange between the atmosphere and metabolising cells, it is understandable that diseases of the cardiovascular system and the lungs result in abnormalities of gas exchange during exercise. A CPET using respiratory gas analysis and a bicycle ergometer will give more relevant information than any history of risk factors or physical examination at rest. The external workload and oxygen consumption are measured accurately during exercise, thus estimates of functional capacity are redundant.

The CPET unit should be an integral part of a preanaesthetic clinic (PAC). It must have sufficient flexibility to perform a test at very short notice, thus preventing repeated visits to the hospital by an already nervous and stressed patient. Our preferred method for preoperative evaluation is a submaximal CPET in which the goal is determination of the anaerobic threshold not maximal aerobic capacity. The AT is an easily measured, repeatable and a volitionally independent measure of functional capacity. It is interesting to note that our discriminator, an AT of 11 ml.kg^{-1}.min^{-1}, is equal to approximately 3 METs, not the 4 METs estimated by the ACC/AHA Guidelines[15] and very different to the 5-MET peak oxygen uptake, the lower limit of accuracy of the DASI.[41] The CPET will accurately determine the severity of functional limitation prior to major surgery. Measurement of the anaerobic threshold 'may provide the best quantitation of the degree of impairment . . . and probably at least cost'.[44]

As previously mentioned, we have shown that cardiovascular mortality is virtually restricted to patients with an AT less than $11 \text{ ml.kg}^{-1}.\text{min}^{-1}$. Analysis of our database for 1480 patients shows a cardiovascular mortality of 22 out of 424 patients with an AT less than $11 \text{ ml.kg}^{-1}.\text{min}^{-1}$. In contrast, cardiovascular mortality was 5 out of 1056 patients with an AT greater than $11 \text{ ml.kg}^{-1}.\text{min}^{-1}$. In percentage terms this represents a mortality rate in the low AT group of 5% compared to 0.5% in the higher AT group, i.e. a ten-fold difference. If the patient, whilst on their medication, has an AT greater than $11 \text{ ml.kg}^{-1}.\text{min}^{-1}$ there is no need to cease or modify it. A problem may arise if the patient has a low AT, revealing a low cardiopulmonary reserve, and is taking potentially negative inotrope medication such as beta-blockade. If this situation arises the dose should be modified, taking into account the risk of postoperative cardiac failure versus the risk of postoperative myocardial ischaemia.

Dosing of beta-blockade appears to vary considerably from one country to another. For example, in Australia, there is little or no attempt to relate dose to body mass index (BMI). We feel individualisation of therapy is a more rational and logical approach than recommendations for universal prescription of beta-blockade or sympatholysis with clonidine based on a history of risk factors.[45] Only a test that objectively and simultaneously evaluates both cardiopulmonary function and myocardial ischaemia will enable a proper risk assessment in this situation.

The ECG stress test: a test for ischaemia not cardiac failure

We feel that current evidence does not support the use of the exercise ECG as a screening test for determination of high risk for major surgery. A meta-analysis of 132 studies of exercise ECGs has shown an average sensitivity of only 68% and a specificity of 77%.[46] To put these figures into perspective and on the basis of these numbers, 32% of patients with myocardial ischaemia will not have a positive exercise ECG test. Further, 23% of patients tested will be characterised as false positive and may have surgery delayed and are likely to have investigations for a disease they do not have. The exercise ECG test concentrates only on myocardial ischaemia which, as we have already pointed out, is not the major problem. In addition it is not possible to objectively measure exercise capacity or oxygen uptake from an exercise ECG study, and the instantaneous estimate of actual work rate is very inaccurate.[21]

In addition to these problems, many 'high cardiac risk' patients may have an ECG that is not interpretable. This includes patients such as those with left bundle branch block, paced rhythm or conduction abnormalities.[40] These do not present a problem for assessment of cardiopulmonary function and functional reserve using submaximal CPET with respiratory gas analysis. Significant information can be gained even if interpretation of the ECG for ischaemic change is not possible.[24] The analysis of gas exchange may be used to identify decreased stroke volume caused by myocardial ischaemia during exercise. With CPET and simple monitoring of heart rate in absence of an interpretable ECG, the question, 'Is the patient able to achieve an acceptable work rate and level of oxygen uptake?' may still be answered. Similarly other contentious issues such as whether or not drugs such as digoxin or beta-blockers should be ceased some time before the test is performed[47] are less of a problem using CPET. The reason for performing the test will influence the decision regarding medications. However, in all our studies using CPET for preoperative evaluation, all patients were tested, as a matter of policy, whilst they continued with all medication.

The 1996 American College of Cardiology and the American Heart Association Guidelines for Preoperative Evaluation of Patients for Non-Cardiac Surgery[48] state that coronary artery disease in the presence of good functional capacity is not a high-risk situation. The ACC/AHA 2002 update[49] specifically states that myocardial ischemia at high levels of exercise is a low-risk situation. They suggest that high levels of exercise are represented by 85% of age-predicted values. This is in keeping with our own findings, which show that myocardial ischaemia occurring late in exercise with an anaerobic threshold exceeding $13\,ml.kg^{-1}.min^{-1}$ is associated with good functional capacity and very low operative risk.[50] Myocardial ischaemia occurring early in exercise is associated with a lower AT (less than $11\,ml.kg^{-1}.min^{-1}$) and a much higher operative risk. This shows the discriminatory value of CPET when combined with temporal analysis of a simultaneous ECG.

Exercise ECG tests performed by cardiologists are almost always performed in patients with a history of chest pain or shortness of breath on exercise. This results in a selection bias in favour of patients testing positive, i.e. tests are performed in a population at risk. If a patient has a positive exercise ECG test this will often result in a series of tests to further evaluate the problem.

Other screening tests

As mentioned above, tests such as dipyridamole–thallium scintigraphy or dobutamine stress echocardiography, whilst of value in diagnosis and management of myocardial ischaemia in the general population, have been shown to be poor screening tests for assessment of cardiac risk before non-cardiac surgery.[2,4] Nevertheless, patients with a history or symptoms and signs of cardiac failure may be investigated by echocardiography or radionuclide ventriculography. Whilst these may be of value in assessment of valvular disease or systolic cardiac failure, they will not identify those patients with predominant diastolic cardiac failure. This is defined in a patient with signs and symptoms of heart failure as a normal ejection fraction and increased left ventricular end-diastolic pressure.[51] As epidemiologic studies have established that 40% to 50% of patients with heart failure have a normal ejection fraction[52,53] this would throw even more doubt on the value of echocardiography or radionuclide ventriculography as a screening test for major surgery.

Preoperative testing does not carry such a heavy bias, as the majority of patients have no cardiac history. Bodenheimer[54] makes the very important point that much of the preoperative invasive testing fails to focus on the real question, 'Can this patient reasonably have non-cardiac surgery?' The only risk factor common to most patients is age; most do not report symptoms of myocardial ischaemia and are otherwise 'healthy' for their age. The intent of a screening test prior to major surgery is to answer the question posed by Bodenheimer, and age as discussed above, is irrelevant.

The new paradigm

Flow chart for perioperative management using CPET

In 1999 we proposed a flow chart for perioperative management of patients for major surgery based on the results of CPET.[19] Analysis of risk factors for coronary artery disease (e.g. diabetes, hypertension, hyperlipidaemia, smoking) had no role in the evaluation. The age and the cardiac history of the patient were used only to identify those patients who required preoperative assessment of functional capacity. Perioperative management was determined by the cardiopulmonary function as measured by CPET and by the surgery-specific risk. This structured approach to perioperative care in patients recognised to be at different degrees of risk allowed resources to be allocated appropriately to each risk group. We reported our results using this system in a series of 548 patients in 1999.[19] No patient triaged to ward management died. There were no unplanned postoperative admissions to the intensive care unit (ICU) from the surgical wards and cardiovascular mortality was confined to patients identified as 'at risk' by CPET. In addition, by using this system we were able to reduce morbidity and mortality and, importantly, reduce ICU resource utilisation and length of ICU stay.

Our management plan has evolved slightly since 1999. The main reason for change is the increasing sophistication of an 'outreach nursing service' (see Chapter 9). Trained intensive care nursing staff follow the progress of patients who have had major surgery even if they are managed on the ward. Problems are then referred to specialists in perioperative medicine, not junior medical staff. The availability of a 24-hour post surgery recovery ward run by anaesthetists further enhances the standard of care of the higher-risk patients. We still recommend that all patients scheduled for major intra-cavity surgery who are over 60 years of age, or any patient younger than 60 years with a history of cardiac failure or myocardial ischaemia, should be evaluated preoperatively by a CPET. This applies to thoracic surgery as well as to abdominal surgery, a point emphasised recently by Gould.[55] In our triage system for postoperative management (Fig. 1.5), patients with an

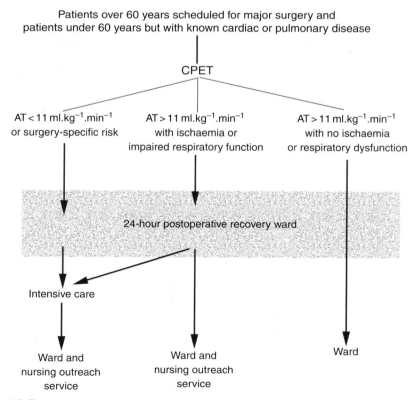

Fig. 1.5 Flow chart for surgical patients using CPET showing management plan based on cardiopulmonary exercise testing and surgery-specific risk.

AT greater than $11\,ml.kg^{-1}.min^{-1}$ and no other abnormalities on CPET are managed by standard care on the general surgical ward. This also applies to patients with an AT greater than $11\,ml.kg^{-1}.min^{-1}$ but with myocardial ischaemia or ventilation perfusion mismatching on CPET. These patients have an acceptable cardiopulmonary reserve but the finding of ischaemia or impaired ventilatory function suggests it would be prudent to have involvement from the 'outreach surgical nurses'. Particular attention would be paid to fluid balance and markers of global perfusion such as plasma lactate and urine volume. Patients with an AT less than $11\,ml.kg^{-1}.min^{-1}$ are at highest risk and should be managed electively in the intensive care unit with invasive monitoring of oxygen-dependent variables, where appropriate, in addition to the perfusion markers above. This is the group of patients in whom the postoperative oxygen demand imposes a severe stress on the cardiopulmonary system. Because of the high surgery-specific risk those patients scheduled for oesophageal or aortic surgery are also monitored postoperatively in this manner, regardless of the result of the CPET. Notwithstanding this, we still test all such patients in the CPET laboratory.

Summary

We believe that concentration on the detection and management of myocardial ischaemia as the risk factor in major non-cardiac surgery is incorrect. We have found that postoperative outcome is influenced mainly by cardiopulmonary function and that postoperative morbidity and mortality following major surgery are mainly caused by a condition we have termed 'postoperative cardiac failure' and not by myocardial ischaemia. We have shown that preoperative identification of patients at risk of postoperative cardiac complications is readily achievable using non-invasive CPET. Further, we have found that modification of perioperative management for such patients, including elective ICU admission and use of haemodynamic monitoring, dramatically lowers morbidity, and results in lower mortality and improved resource utilisation.

References

1. Sprague H. The heart in surgery: analysis of the results in surgery on cardiac patients during the past ten years at the Massachusetts General Hospital. *Surg Gynecol Obstet* 1929; 49: 54–8.
2. Mangano DT, London MJ, Tubau JF, *et al*. Dipyridamole thallium-201 scintigraphy as a preoperative screening test. A reexamination of its predictive potential. Study of Perioperative Ischemia Research Group. *Circulation* 1991; 84: 493–502.
3. Mantha S, Roizen MF, Barnard J, *et al*. Relative effectiveness of four preoperative tests for predicting adverse cardiac outcomes after vascular surgery: a meta-analysis. *Anesth Analg* 1994; 79: 422–33.

4. Halm EA, Browner WS, Tubau JF, *et al*. Echocardiography for assessing cardiac risk in patients having noncardiac surgery. Study of Perioperative Ischemia Research Group. *Ann Intern Med* 1996; **125**: 433–41.
5. Hollenberg SM. Preoperative cardiac risk assessment. *Chest* 1999; 115:51S–7S.
6. Mangano DT, Layug EL, Wallace A, *et al*. Effect of atenolol on mortality and cardiovascular morbidity after noncardiac surgery. Multicenter Study of Perioperative Ischemia Research Group. *N Engl J Med* 1996; **335**: 1713–20.
7. Poldermans D, Boersma E, Bax JJ, *et al*. The effect of bisoprolol on perioperative mortality and myocardial infarction in high-risk patients undergoing vascular surgery. Dutch Echocardiographic Cardiac Risk Evaluation Applying Stress Echocardiography Study Group. *N Engl J Med* 1999; **341**: 1789–94.
8. London MJ, Zaugg M, Schaub MC, *et al*. Perioperative beta-adrenergic receptor blockade: physiologic foundations and clinical controversies. *Anesthesiology* 2004; **100**: 170–5.
9. Devereaux PJ, Beattie WS, Choi PT, *et al*. How strong is the evidence for the use of perioperative beta blockers in non-cardiac surgery? Systematic review and meta-analysis of randomised controlled trials. *BMJ* 2005; **331**: 313–21.
10. Yeager MP, Fillinger MP, Hettleman BD, *et al*. Perioperative beta-blockade and late cardiac outcomes: a complementary hypothesis. *J Cardiothorac Vasc Anesth* 2005; **19**: 237–41.
11. Wetterslev J, Juul A. Benefits and harms of perioperative beta-blockade. *Best Pract Res Clin Anaesthesiol* 2006; **20**: 285–302.
12. Fleisher LA. Perioperative myocardial ischemia and infarction. *Int Anesthesiol Clin* 1992; **30**: 1–17.
13. Aitkenhead AR. Cardiac morbidity after non-cardiac surgery. *Lancet* 1993; **341**: 731–2.
14. Kertai MD, Bax JJ, Klein J, *et al*. Is there any reason to withhold beta blockers from high-risk patients with coronary artery disease during surgery? *Anesthesiology* 2004; **100**: 4–7.
15. Eagle KA, Berger PB, Calkins H, *et al*. ACC/AHA guideline update for perioperative cardiovascular evaluation for noncardiac surgery – executive summary: a report of the American College of Cardiology/American Heart Association Task Force on Practice Guidelines (Committee to Update the 1996 Guidelines on Perioperative Cardiovascular Evaluation for Noncardiac Surgery). *Circulation* 2002; **105**: 1257–67.
16. Older P, Smith R, Hall A, *et al*. Preoperative cardiopulmonary risk assessment by cardiopulmonary exercise testing. *Crit Care Resusc* 2000; **2**: 198–208.
17. Goto T, Takase H, Toriyama T, *et al*. Circulating concentrations of cardiac proteins indicate the severity of congestive heart failure. *Heart* 2003; **89**: 1303–7.
18. Ammann P, Pfisterer M, Fehr T, *et al*. Raised cardiac troponins. *BMJ* 2004; **328**: 1028–9.
19. Older P, Hall A, Hader R. Cardiopulmonary exercise testing as a screening test for perioperative management of major surgery in the elderly. *Chest* 1999; **116**: 355–62.
20. Older P, Smith R, Courtney P, *et al*. Preoperative evaluation of cardiac failure and ischemia in elderly patients by cardiopulmonary exercise testing. *Chest* 1993; **104**: 701–4.

21. Wasserman K, Hansen JE, Sue DY, *et al. Principles of Exercise Testing and Interpretation*. Second edn. Philadelphia, PA: Lea & Febiger, 1994.
22. Beaver WL, Wasserman K, Whipp BJ. A new method for detecting anaerobic threshold by gas exchange. *J Appl Physiol* 1986; **60**: 2020–7.
23. Weber KT, Janicki JS. Cardiopulmonary exercise testing for evaluation of chronic cardiac failure. *Am J Cardiol* 1985; **55**: 22A–31A.
24. Belardinelli R, Lacalaprice F, Carle F, *et al.* Exercise-induced myocardial ischaemia detected by cardiopulmonary exercise testing. *Eur Heart J* 2003; **24**: 1304–13.
25. Older P, Hall A. The role of cardiopulmonary exercise testing for preoperative evaluation of the elderly. In Wasserman K, ed. *Exercise Gas Exchange in Heart Disease*. Armonk, NY: Futura Publishing Company, 1996; pp. 287–97.
26. Mangano DT. Perioperative cardiac morbidity. *Anesthesiology* 1990; **72**: 153–84.
27. Raby KE, Goldman L, Creager MA, *et al.* Correlation between preoperative ischemia and major cardiac events after peripheral vascular surgery. *N Engl J Med* 1989; **321**: 1296–300.
28. Urban MK, Markowitz SM, Gordon MA, *et al.* Postoperative prophylactic administration of beta-adrenergic blockers in patients at risk for myocardial ischemia. *Anesth Analg* 2000; **90**: 1257–61.
29. Abhayaratna WP, Smith WT, Becker NG, *et al.* Prevalence of heart failure and systolic ventricular dysfunction in older Australians: the Canberra Heart Study. *Med J Aust* 2006; **184**: 151–4.
30. Clark RA, McLennan S, Dawson A, *et al.* Uncovering a hidden epidemic: a study of the current burden of heart failure in Australia. *Heart Lung Circ* 2004; **13**: 266–73.
31. Hernandez AF, Whellan DJ, Stroud S, *et al.* Outcomes in heart failure patients after major noncardiac surgery. *J Am Coll Cardiol* 2004; **44**: 1446–53.
32. Dunselman PH, Kuntze CE, van Bruggen A, *et al.* Value of New York Heart Association classification, radionuclide ventriculography, and cardiopulmonary exercise tests for selection of patients for congestive heart failure studies. *Am Heart J* 1988; **116**: 1475–82.
33. Wasserman K. Preoperative evaluation of cardiovascular reserve in the elderly. *Chest* 1993; **104**: 663–4.
34. Lavoisier A-L. *Traite elementaire de Chimie*. First edn. Paris, 1790; Dover edn. 1965.
35. Myers J, Prakash M, Froelicher V, *et al.* Exercise capacity and mortality among men referred for exercise testing. *N Engl J Med* 2002; **346**: 793–801.
36. Gerson MC, Hurst JM, Hertzberg VS, *et al.* Cardiac prognosis in noncardiac geriatric surgery. *Ann Intern Med* 1985; **103**: 832–7.
37. Greenburg AG, Saik RP, Pridham D. Influence of age on mortality of colon surgery. *Am J Surg* 1985; **150**: 65–70.
38. Gitt AK, Wasserman K, Kilkowski C, *et al.* Exercise anaerobic threshold and ventilatory efficiency identify heart failure patients for high risk of early death. *Circulation* 2002; **106**: 3079–84.
39. Gibbons RJ, Balady GJ, Timothy Bricker J, *et al.* ACC/AHA 2002 guideline update for exercise testing: summary article. A report of the American College of Cardiology/American Heart Association Task Force on Practice Guidelines (Committee to Update the 1997 Exercise Testing Guidelines). *J Am Coll Cardiol* 2002; **40**: 1531–40.

40. Hlatky MA, Boineau RE, Higginbotham MB, *et al*. A brief self-administered questionnaire to determine functional capacity (the Duke Activity Status Index). *Am J Cardiol* 1989; **64**: 651–4.

41. Carliner NH, Fisher ML, Plotnick GD, *et al*. Routine preoperative exercise testing in patients undergoing major noncardiac surgery. *Am J Cardiol* 1985; **56**: 51–8.

42. McPhail N, Calvin JE, Shariatmadar A, *et al*. The use of preoperative exercise testing to predict cardiac complications after arterial reconstruction. *J Vasc Surg* 1988; **7**: 60–8.

43. Froelicher V. Interpretation of specific exercise test responses. In: Froelicher V, ed. *Exercise and the Heart*. Chicago, IL: Year Book Medical Publishers, 1987; pp. 83–145.

44. Wasserman K. Diagnosing cardiovascular and lung pathophysiology from exercise gas exchange. *Chest* 1997; **112**: 1091–101.

45. Wallace A. *Perioperative Cardiac Risk Reduction Therapy*; www.cardiacengineering.com.

46. Lee TH, Boucher CA. Clinical practice. Noninvasive tests in patients with stable coronary artery disease. *N Engl J Med* 2001; **344**: 1840–5.

47. Grecu L, Mehaffey C, Isselbacher E. Preoperative noninvasive cardiac testing: which test and why? *Int Anesthesiol Clin* 2002; **40**: 121–32.

48. Eagle K, Brunage B, Chaitman B, *et al*. Guidelines for perioperative cardiovascular evaluation for noncardiac surgery. Report of the American College of Cardiology/American Heart Association Task Force on Practise Guidelines. Committee on Perioperative Cardiovascular Evaluation for Non-cardiac Surgery. *Circulation* 1996; **93**: 1278–317.

49. Eagle KA, Berger PB, Calkins H, *et al*. ACC/AHA guideline update for perioperative cardiovascular evaluation for noncardiac surgery – executive summary. A report of the American College of Cardiology/American Heart Association Task Force on Practice Guidelines (Committee to Update the 1996 Guidelines on Perioperative Cardiovascular Evaluation for Noncardiac Surgery). *Anesth Analg* 2002; **94**: 1052–64.

50. Older P, Hall A. The role of cardiopulmonary exercise testing in evaluation of surgical patients. In Wasserman K, ed. *Preoperative Assessment of Elderly Surgical Patients*. Armonk, NY: Futura Publishing Company Inc., 2002; pp. 119–33.

51. Zile MR, Baicu CF, Gaasch WH. Diastolic heart failure – abnormalities in active relaxation and passive stiffness of the left ventricle. *N Engl J Med* 2004; **350**: 1953–9.

52. Redfield MM. Understanding "diastolic" heart failure. *N Engl J Med* 2004; **350**: 1930–1.

53. Tresch DD, McGough MF. Heart failure with normal systolic function: a common disorder in older people. *J Am Geriatr Soc* 1995; **43**: 1035–42.

54. Bodenheimer MM. Noncardiac surgery in the cardiac patient: what is the question? *Ann Intern Med* 1996; **124**: 763–6.

55. Gould G, Pearce A. Assessment of suitability for lung resection. *Contin Educ Anaesth, Crit Care Pain* 2006; **6**: 97–100.

Kathleen M. Sherry

Oesophagectomy for cancer

Carcinoma of the oesophagus accounts for 7% of all gastrointestinal malignancies, but there are wide geographical variations in its incidence. In the Western world the incidence of oesophageal carcinoma, particularly adenocarcinoma, has been increasing over the past 30 years and the current rate is approximately 10 per 100 000, of which 5 per 100 000 is adenocarcinoma. Adenocarcinoma is more frequent in Caucasians and squamous cell carcinoma is more frequent in those of African descent. Worldwide the highest incidence of oesophageal carcinoma is in parts of China and northern Iran where the rate is up to 170 per 100 000, most of which are of squamous cell type. Regional differences have been linked to factors such as nitrosamine food preservatives and alcohol consumption. Oesophageal cancer increases with age and the median age at presentation is 70 years. Males more commonly develop adenocarcinoma than females by a ratio of 7:1, and the male to female ratio for all oesophageal cancer is 2:1.

The main risk factors for the development of oesophageal cancer are alcohol and cigarette smoking, which have a synergistic effect for squamous cell carcinoma.[1] Chronic inflammation and stasis, for example, caustic stricture and achalasia, increase the risk for squamous cell carcinoma, as does coeliac disease, Plummer–Vinson syndrome and tylosis (hereditary hyperkeratosis of the palms and soles). Adenocarcinoma is associated with Barrett's oesophagus and the increase in adenocarcinoma in the Western world may be related to an increase in obesity, leading to a high incidence of gastro-oesophageal reflux disease.[2,3] Patients of lower socioeconomic groups are more likely to develop oesophageal cancer[4] and this may be related to deficiencies of vitamins A and C and trace elements.

Recent Advances in Anaesthesia and Intensive Care 24, ed. J. N. Cashman and R. M. Grounds.
Published by Cambridge University Press. © Cambridge University Press 2007.

Tumours tend to occur in areas of oesophageal narrowing and these are the pharyngo–oesophageal junction, the junction of the upper and middle third, and the lower oesophagus where it passes through the diaphragm. Carcinoma in the upper two-thirds of the oesophagus is of squamous cell type and 90% of those in the lower third are adenocarcinoma arising in a region of specialised columnar epithelial metaplasia. Patients commonly present with dysphagia and weight loss but may also complain of regurgitation or respiratory symptoms from overspill. At the time of presentation most patients will have locally invasive disease or metastases and only 30–50% will have a disease stage that is potentially surgically curative. Open surgery for oesophagectomy may be trans-hiatal or trans-thoracic. The trans-hiatal and left thoracoabdominal approaches are suitable for adenocarcinomas in the lower third of the oesophagus, but for higher lesions the two stage Ivor–Lewis with a right thoracotomy is indicated.[5] Results of oesphagectomy for cancer are poor with a 30-day mortality of approximately 10% and fewer than 30% of patients survive more than five years. There is wide variation in postoperative mortality between centres with reports ranging from over 20% to under 5%. There is also evidence that high-volume centres have lower postoperative mortality[6,7,8,9] and better long-term results.[10] The definition of high volume varies and some studies have arbitrarily defined it as seven or more cases each year but Metzger and colleagues[10] in an analysis of 13 papers concluded that 20 or more cases per year was more closely linked to improved postoperative outcome. Several studies have shown that operative mortality rates following oesophagectomy are falling.[6,10] Dimick and colleagues[6] used the United States Nationwide Inpatient Sample data to show that between 1988 and 2000 operative mortality decreased from 11% to 7.5% in high-volume hospitals but was unchanged in low-volume hospitals performing six or fewer operations each year. The reasons for improved results are not entirely clear but are likely to include patient selection,[11,12] neoadjuvant chemoradiation,[12] the experience of the surgeon[13,14,15,16,17] and multidiscipline teamwork. Referral patterns are now changing, with more operations being performed at high-volume hospitals.[6,11]

Preoperative risk assessment

The incidence of postoperative complications following oesophagectomy is high, and understanding preoperative risk factors for postoperative morbidity and mortality can be used to stratify patients according to risk and influence the preoperative investigation and the level of perioperative care. Rindani and colleagues[18] analysed all papers published in English between 1986–96 that reported complications for trans-hiatal oesophagectomy (THO) or Ivor–Lewis oesophagectomy (ILO). The operative mortality for

Table 2.1 Complications following oesophagectomy.[18]

	Trans-hiatal no. (%)	Ivor–Lewis oesophagec-tomy no. (%)
Pulmonary	557/2329 (24)	475/1904 (25)
Respiratory failure	86	75
Pneumonia	302	341
Pleural effusion	33	10
Empyema	15	47
Pneumothorax	121	6
Cardiac	224/1806 (12.4)	153/1459 (10.5)
Chylothorax	26/1217 (2.1)	43/1271 (3.4)
Intrathoracic bleed	40/813 (4.9)	46/921 (5)
Wound infection	100/1138 (8.8)	78/1267 (6.2)
Anastomotic leak	372/2329 (16)	190/1907 (10)
Anastomotic stricture	476/1647 (28)	215/1366 (16)
Recurrent laryngeal palsy	197/1753 (11.2)	74/1552 (4.8)

THO was 6.3%, compared with 9.5% for ILO. Five-year survival was comparable at 24% for THO and 26% for ILO. However, if patients who had undergone adjuvant treatment were excluded from analysis the five-year survival was 25% for THO compared with 35% for ILO. A summary of the complications is presented in Table 2.1.

Respiratory complications occur in about 1 in 4 patients and are the main cause of postoperative morbidity and death. This is followed by cardiac complications, including myocardial infarction and arrhythmia, and anastomotic leak. Preoperative predictors of respiratory complications include preoperative pulmonary dysfunction[19,20,21,22,23,24,25] and a history of smoking.[26] Other factors predicting postoperative complications include age,[21,22,23,24,27,28,29] liver impairment,[20,23,25] poor physiological or performance status,[20,23,24,28] nutritional deficiency,[30] renal impairment[23] and diabetes.[23] In the 1990s there was an increase in the use of neoadjuvant chemoradiotherapy with recognition that a good response to neoadjuvant treatment can improve the cancer stage and patient survival.[31] There are concerns that preoperative chemoradiotherapy can increase perioperative morbidity and mortality,[31,32] and this appears to be so for those who develop high-grade toxicity reactions to chemotherapy or receive a radiotherapy dose sufficient to affect their lung function[33] and performance status.[34,35]

In 2002 the Association of Upper Gastrointestinal Surgeons, British Society of Gastroenterology and British Association of Surgical Oncology produced guidelines for the management of oesophageal and gastric cancer.[5] They emphasised that the patient's physiological status is an important factor in determining the outcome of major surgery, and a detailed medical history and examination directed towards detecting co-morbidities is mandatory. Particularly common co-morbidities in patients with oesophageal cancer are ischaemic heart disease, respiratory disease, anaemia or polycythaemia, hypoalbuminaemia, liver impairment and immunodeficiency. As part of their work-up patients with co-morbidities need preoperative referral to specialist physicians to optimise their medical treatment. The incidence of ischaemic heart disease, including silent myocardial ischaemia, is likely to be high and may be present in up to 25% of patients[36,37] so the involvement within the team of a cardiologist with experience of minimising perioperative risk from ischaemic heart disease is important.

Scoring systems

In 1992 Bartels and colleagues[20] devised a scoring system specifically to assist risk stratification of oesophagectomy patients. They reviewed 432 patients who had undergone oesophagectomy in their centre between 1982 and 1991 and evaluated their preoperative physiological parameters in order to determine those that correlated with the postoperative course. They found that pulmonary, hepatic and cardiac function and general status were most closely linked to postoperative risk. General status was assessed using the Karnofsky Performance Scale Index, which classifies cancer patients according to their functional impairment (see Table 2.2). The four parameters of pulmonary, cardiac and hepatic function and general status were ascribed weighting values, and for each patient these four parameters were graded according to the severity of the condition as normal $= 1$, compromised $= 2$ or severely impaired $= 3$ (see Table 2.3). The grade for each parameter was multiplied by its weighting and the sum of these scores used to determine risk. Three risk groups were identified. Low risk, 11–15 points ($n = 166$), 3.6% 30-day mortality; medium risk, 16–21 points ($n = 194$), 8.7% 30-day mortality; and high risk, 22–33 points ($n = 72$), 28% 30-day mortality. The validity of this scoring system was tested prospectively on 121 patients in their centre and subsequently the inclusion of the composite score into the process of patient selection and choice of the procedure resulted in a decrease of postoperative mortality rate from 9.4% to 1.6%.

In 2000 Furguson and Durkin[22] devised a scoring system to predict pulmonary complications after oesophagectomy for cancer. They analysed retrospective data from case notes for oesophagectomy operations between 1980 and 1989, and information from their surgical database for oesophagectomies from 1990 onwards. Multivariable logistic regression analysis was performed on data from 220 patients. This indicated that at age greater than 50 years, FEV_1 (forced expiratory volume in one second) was $< 90\%$

Table 2.2 Karnofsky Performance Status Scale Definitions for Rating (%) Criteria.

Able to carry on normal activity and to work; no special care needed.	100%	Normal and with no complaints; no evidence of disease.
	90%	Able to carry on normal activity; minor signs or symptoms of disease.
	80%	Normal activity with effort; some signs or symptoms of disease.
Unable to work; able to live at home and care for most personal needs; varying amount of assistance needed.	70%	Cares for self but is unable to carry on normal activity or to do active work.
	60%	Requires occasional assistance, but is able to care for most of his/her personal needs.
	50%	Requires considerable assistance and frequent medical care.
Unable to care for self; requires equivalent of institutional or hospital care; disease may be progressing rapidly.	40%	Disabled; requires special care and assistance.
	30%	Severely disabled; hospital admission is indicated although death is not imminent.
	20%	Very sick; hospital admission necessary; active supportive treatment necessary.
	10%	Moribund; fatal processes progressing rapidly.
	0%	Dead

of predicted and the Eastern Cooperative oncology Group Performance Status, a five-point scale similar to the Karnofsky Index, could be used as a basis for a scoring system. On testing the scoring system in their unit they found it had a limited ability to predict cardiovascular and cardiopulmonary complications and could not predict mortality.

Although scoring systems can be useful they need to be tested and validated in a population other than that in which they are devised. Zafirellis and colleagues[38] demonstrated the importance of testing scoring systems. They assessed the accuracy of the Physiological and Operative Severity Score for the enUmeration of Mortality and morbidity (POSSUM) to predict mortality and morbidity in 213 patients with oesophageal cancer who underwent surgery in their unit between 1990 and 1999. The POSSUM scoring system was initially devised as an audit tool to allow risk adjustment for the physical status of patients undergoing a range of general surgical operations, but it has often been used by clinicians for surgical sub-specialties.[39] Zafirellis and colleagues found that the original POSSUM scoring over-predicted mortality and morbidity rates for oesophagectomy patients. They concluded that the POSSUM scoring system would need modification with

Table 2.3 Bartel's scoring system for operative risk assessment of patients with oesophageal cancer.

Function (weighting)	Finding	Value
Pulmonary (2)		
1 = Normal	VC > 90% **and** PaO$_2$ > 70 mmHg	2
2 = Compromised	VC < 90% **or** PaO$_2$ < 70 mmHg	4
3 = Severely impaired	VC < 90% **and** PaO$_2$ < 70 mmHg	6
Hepatic function (2)		
1 = Normal	ABT > 0.4 (2.4%)	2
2 = Compromised	ABT < 0.4, no cirrhosis	4
3 = Severely impaired	Cirrhosis	6
Cardiac function by cardiology opinion (3)		
1 = Normal	Normal risk for major surgical procedure	3
2 = Compromised	Intermediate risk for major surgical procedure	6
3 = Severely impaired	High risk for major surgical procedure	9
General status (4)		
1 = Normal	Karnofsky index > 80% **and** good co-operation	4
2 = Compromised	Karnofsky index < 80% **or** poor co-operation	8
3 = Severely impaired	Karnofsky index < 80% **and** poor co-operation	12

ABT = aminopyrine breath test; VC = vital capacity; PaO$_2$ = arterial partial pressure of oxygen. The weighting is in brackets after each function. Thus if a patient has severely impaired hepatic function this scores as a severity of 3, multiplied by the weighting for hepatic function which is 2; thus hepatic function in that patient scores 6 (the sum in the value column). For an individual patient, if the value for each of the four functions is summed up, then an overall score (value) for that patient can be obtained.

the introduction of further physiological variables to make it a valuable tool. In 2004 Tekkis and colleagues[40] modified the POSSUM scoring system to create O-POSSUM (O = oesophagogastric), which is specifically weighted for upper gastrointestinal surgery and incorporates the operation and disease stage. This was devised using data from 1042 patients undergoing oesophageal ($n = 538$) or gastric ($n = 504$) surgery between 1994 and 2000. Using the area under the receiver–operator characteristic curve there was higher discrimination using the O-POSSUM (79.7% versus 74.3% for the P-POSSUM; P = Portsmouth). The O-POSSUM scoring system looks promising but to date the only other population it has been evaluated in is 126 patients undergoing elective gastric surgery.[41] A web-based calculator for the O-POSSUM scoring system is available (http://www.riskprediction. org.uk/op-index.php).

Preoperative investigation

The minimum preoperative investigations for oesophagectomy include haematology and biochemistry profiles, arterial blood gases and pulmonary function tests, resting electrocardiogram (ECG) and chest x-ray. In

---

Table 2.4 Duke Activity Status Index.

Can you:

1. Take care of yourself – that is eating, dressing, bathing or using the toilet?
2. Walk indoors, such as around the house?
3. Walk a block or two on level ground?
4. Climb a flight of stairs or walk up a hill?
5. Run a short distance?
6. Do light work around the house like dusting or washing dishes?
7. Do moderate activity around the house like vacuuming, sweeping floors or carrying in groceries?
8. Do heavy work around the house like scrubbing floors or moving heavy furniture?
9. Do yardwork like raking leaves, weeding or pushing a power mower?
10. Have sexual relations?
11. Participate in moderate recreational activities such as golf, bowling, dancing, doubles tennis, throwing a baseball or football?
12. Participate in strenuous sport such as swimming, singles tennis, football, basketball or skiing?

---

recent years increasing attention has been paid to assessing integrated cardiopulmonary functional capacity. Oxygen consumption at rest is $3.5\,\mathrm{ml.kg^{-1}.min^{-1}}$ but with the surgical stress following oesophagectomy this will increase to perhaps 6 to $7\,\mathrm{ml.kg^{-1}.min^{-1}}$ at rest, and higher on mobilisation or if complications supervene. In order to determine whether a patient can deliver sufficient oxygen for this consumption they need some form of cardiopulmonary assessment. The most basic assessment is that of their preoperative exercise capacity. The Duke Activity Status Index[42] is an estimate of energy requirements for various activities based on metabolic equivalents (METs), where oxygen consumption at rest is 1 MET. Table 2.4 shows examples of activities, and for major surgery the patient will need to achieve an oxygen consumption of $14\,\mathrm{ml.kg^{-1}.min^{-1}}$ or activity greater than 4 METs, that is the ability to climb one flight of stairs without stopping.

In the early 1980s, when pulse oximetry became widely available, the ability to climb a flight of stairs without desaturating more than 4% was used as a quick and convenient way of assessing patients' cardiopulmonary reserve. In the early 1990s this was more formalised in the incremental shuttle-walk test, which is how far the subject can walk when walking at a predetermined increasing speed between cones placed 10 m apart. In the test there are 12 levels each of 1-minute duration with walking speeds that rise incrementally from 1.2 miles per hour (1.9 km per hour) to 5.3 miles per hour (8.5 km per hour). Achieving less than 250 m indicates maximum oxygen consumption ($\dot{V}O_2$ max) of less than $10\,\mathrm{ml.kg^{-1}.min^{-1}}$ and very high risk. Achieving between 250–450 m indicates increased risk, and

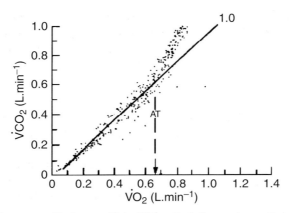

Fig. 2.1 From Wasserman, K., Beaver, W. L., Whipp, B. J. Gas exchange theory and the lactic acidosis (anaerobic) threshold. *Circulation* 1990; **81**(Suppl. II):S14–S30.

greater than 450 m indicates a $\dot{V}O_2$ max of greater than $14\,ml.kg^{-1}.min^{-1}$ and low risk. Desaturation on pulse oximetry of greater than 4% during the test indicates increased risk, as does myocardial ischaemia on Holter monitoring. There are several other forms of timed walking tests – for example, the 6-minute walking test, which is the maximum distance a patient can walk in six minutes. These types of cardiopulmonary functional capacity tests are limited in that they do not have good reproducibility and are dependent on motivation.

In 1988 Older and colleagues started using more formal cardiopulmonary exercise testing to identify high-risk patients for major surgery.[37] Cardiopulmonary exercise testing involves the use of respiratory gas analysis and continuous ECG monitoring (see Chapter 1). Older and colleagues use the anaerobic threshold (AT) as the end point. At rest a subject will consume about $250\,ml.min^{-1}$ oxygen (O_2) and produce $200\,ml.min^{-1}$ carbon dioxide (CO_2) giving a respiratory quotient (CO_2/O_2) of 0.8. With increasing exercise the O_2 consumption ($\dot{V}O_2$) will increase in line with CO_2 production ($\dot{V}CO_2$) until the subject switches to anaerobic metabolism, when CO_2 production will start to rise more quickly than O_2 consumption and the respiratory quotient will exceed 1.0. If $\dot{V}CO_2$ is plotted against $\dot{V}O_2$, the oxygen consumption at AT can be determined at the inflexion point on the V-slope plot (see Fig. 2.1).

Older and colleagues determined that patients with $AT < 11\,ml.kg^{-1}.min^{-1}$ undergoing major surgery were at higher risk of a cardiovascular death, which was compounded if they developed myocardial ischaemia before reaching AT, and they should receive ICU care postoperatively.

Patients who developed myocardial ischaemia after reaching AT are at increased risk compared to those without myocardial ischaemia. In the opinion of the authors the use of AT is preferred as the end point because it is independent of motivation and occurs before maximum aerobic capacity is achieved.

Nagamatsu and colleagues[43] undertook lung function and cardiopulmonary exercise testing in 91 patients undergoing cervicothoracoabdominal oesophagectomy with 3-field lymphadenectomy. The results of these tests were divided by body surface area to minimise differences in physique. Based on outcome, patients were divided into two groups: those who suffered cardiopulmonary complications ($n = 17$) and those who did not ($n = 74$). On multiple logistic regressions analysis of the results of their patients' lung function and cardiopulmonary exercise testing, the authors found that only $\dot{V}O_2$ max.m^{-2} was associated with outcome and that lung function and AT.m^{-2} were not. They then calculated the rate of cardiopulmonary complications based on $\dot{V}O_2$ max.m^{-2}. Cardiopulminary complications occurred in 86% of patients with $\dot{V}O_2$ max.m$^{-2} < 699$ ml.min^{-1}.m^{-2}, 44% of those with $\dot{V}O_2$ max.m^{-2} 700–799 ml.min^{-1}.m^{-2}, 10% of those with $\dot{V}O_2$ max.m^{-2} 800–1099 ml.min^{-1}.m^{-2} and none with $\dot{V}O_2$ max.m$^{-2} > 1100$ ml.min^{-1}.m^{-2}. The authors concluded that postoperative cardiopulmonary complications could not be determined by routine pulmonary function tests alone and that a $\dot{V}O_2$ max.m^{-2} of > 800 ml.min^{-1}.m^{-2} is required for curative transthoracic oesophagectomy. They thought that AT did not correlate with outcome because the metabolic demands for oesophagectomy require cardiopulmonary reserve at higher workloads than for other major surgery. The $\dot{V}O_2$ max is dependent on motivation and they considered that it also indicated mental fitness for the operation.

It is apparent that patients undergoing oesophagectomy for cancer require a multidisciplinary approach. It is clear that high-risk patients who have been identified from their history and basic investigations, particularly if they are of advanced age, have cardiac disease or impaired pulmonary function tests, require an accurate assessment including cardiopulmonary exercise testing. Cardiopulmonary exercise testing before major surgery is currently being investigated in several UK centers. Intensive care physicians and anaesthetists using compact bicycle or arm cycle ergonometers are mainly undertaking this. However, many pulmonary function laboratories also perform cardiopulmonary exercise tests using treadmill equipment. The patients of concern are those with AT < 11 ml.kg^{-1}.min^{-1}, $\dot{V}O_2$ max.m^{-2} of < 800 ml.min^{-1}.m^{-2} and evidence of myocardial ischaemia. Patients falling into this category will need more intensive perioperative care.

Operative care

Operative risk factors for morbidity or mortality include the stage[25] and site of the lesion with more proximal tumours having greater risk,[21,27] the duration of the operation[23,26,27] and duration of one-lung ventilation,[26] haemodynamic instability with fluid, blood and inotropic support requirements,[23,26,27,28] perioperative hypoxaemia[26] and postoperative atrial fibrillation.[44]

It is axiomatic that patients undergoing oesophagectomy need intensive monitoring and meticulous care during their operation with particular attention to fluid management and oxygenation. All should have minimal monitoring, temperature, arterial, central venous and urine output monitoring. Those at high risk also require some form of cardiac output monitoring. Several studies have shown that for major surgery, optimisation of oxygen delivery using fluid and inotropic drugs can improve postoperative outcome. In 1993 Boyd and colleagues[45] randomised 107 high-risk surgical patients to one of two groups: those who underwent standard perioperative care and those who received a dopexamine infusion to increase oxygen delivery to greater than $600 \, ml.min^{-1}.m^{-2}$. They showed that the dopexamine group achieved a 75% reduction in mortality and a 50% reduction in the mean number of complications per patient compared to the control group. In 1999 Wilson and colleagues compared preoperative optimisation of oxygen delivery with dopexamine and with adrenaline.[46] They showed dopexamine to be superior to adrenaline at reducing morbidity, although not mortality. Dopexamine has advantages over dobutamine, and presumably other catecholamines, for patients with ischaemic heart disease as it is less likely to cause myocardial ischaemia.[47] This is because dopexamine predominantly acts at the vasodilatory β_2 adrenoreceptors and DA1 receptors so the increase in cardiac output is achieved mainly by increasing heart rate and stroke volume without greatly increasing stroke work and oxygen demand; however, tachycardia may be a limiting factor. There have been no comparisons between dopexamine and either PDE (phosphodiesterase) inhibitors or calcium sensitisers, which also increase cardiac output without increasing myocardial ischaemia. Dopexamine has other potential benefits in that it should improve hepatic, renal and splanchnic blood flows and so reduce renal ischaemic damage and anastomotic breakdown. There is some clinical evidence that it does improve gastric pH but it should be started early, before any ischaemic insult occurs, and continued for at least six hours.[48] Dopexamine also has some anti-inflammatory properties[49] and may modulate the systemic inflammatory response syndrome (SIRS). The studies on optimising oxygen delivery before major surgery have required patients to be admitted to a high-dependency or intensive care area for some hours before surgery. In many units this is not practical and optimisation of oxygen delivery has to be undertaken during the operation. An observational study by Kusano and colleagues[50] showed that after oesophagectomy oxygen delivery lower than 445 ml.min^{-1}.m^{-2} was associated with increased mortality and that those who developed either anastomotic leak or pneumonia had a significantly lower oxygen delivery than those who did not at six hours after operation. This indicates that high-risk patients, those with co-morbidity, need postoperative high-dependency or intensive care management and ongoing optimisation of oxygen delivery for the first six to 12 hours.

There is increasing evidence that anaesthesia for major thoracoabdominal surgery should include epidural anaesthesia. To assess the quality of pain relief from epidural analgesia Block and colleagues[51] performed a meta-analysis on 100 randomised studies that compared epidural analgesia with parenteral opioid analgesia. When all types of surgery were assessed, epidural analgesia provided significantly better postoperative analgesia than parenteral opioids for the first four days after operation. For thoracic surgery (27 studies) epidural analgesia provided superior analgesia than parenteral opioid, irrespective of whether the epidural included local anaesthetic, with or without opioid, or used opioid alone. However for pain at rest thoracic epidural analgesia (TEA) that included local anaesthetic was better that thoracic or lumbar epidural using opioid alone. To assess the effect of epidural analgesia on outcome Rodgers and colleagues[52] performed a meta-analysis of 141 studies (9559 patients) that reported the effect of neuraxial blockade on morbidity and mortality across all surgical specialties. They concluded that mortality and morbidity across all surgical groups were reduced when neuraxial blockade was used, either alone or as combined with general anaesthesia, however there was insufficient power for sub-group analysis. There are theoretical reasons why thoracic epidural analgesia may be beneficial during and after oesophagogastrectomy. Thoracic epidural analgesia with local anaesthetics can block the cardiac sympathetic innervation, which comes from T_1–T_5. Sympathetic blockade will reduce myocardial oxygen demand and coronary vasoconstriction and so may reduce adverse cardiac events. It has been shown in upper abdominal surgery that epidural analgesia can reduce myocardial ischaemia intraoperatively and postoperatively for the first 24 hours,[53] although this study was not sufficiently powered to show an impact on cardiac morbidity or mortality. However, it has been shown that following thoracic surgery myocardial ischaemia is associated with adverse outcome, but not necessarily primary cardiac events.[36] It is probable that patients with myocardial ischaemia are more likely to succumb to any complications including respiratory complications and sepsis. It is also possible that the vasodilator effects of epidural anaesthesia can reduce the incidence of postoperative heart failure in high-risk surgical patients [54] but recent advances in the treatment of chronic heart failure using the new vasodilator drugs make postoperative heart failure a much lesser problem. The sympathetic block-ade by epidural anaesthesia can modify the postoperative hypercoagulabi-lity state and may decrease the risk of venous thromboembolism. This has been shown in orthopaedic surgery but there is limited data to substantiate an effect in general surgery patients.[52] Epidural anaesthesia appears to be the most effective means of reducing postoperative ileus[55] and may be of specific benefit to patients undergoing oesophagectomy.

Acute lung injury – that is bilateral infiltrates on chest x-ray with pulmonary capillary wedge pressure < 18 mmHg or no evidence of heart failure – may occur in up to 50% of patients following oesophagectomy[56] and in some this will progress to respiratory failure or acute respiratory distress syndrome (ARDS). The causes of acute lung injury after oesophagectomy are similar to those following lung resection. Surgery causes direct trauma to intrathoracic structures including the lung and lymphatic drainage, and damage to the thoracic duct following oesophagectomy is well recognised.[18] During one-lung ventilation the ventilated lung is often subjected to hyperoxia to com-pensate for intrapulmonary shunting, high inflation pressures and volume trauma, all of which may contribute to lung damage.[57] The non-ventilated lung is susceptible to ischaemia/reperfusion injury[57] with the consequent release of pro-inflammatory mediators. An increase of pro-inflammatory mediators in blood and bronchoalveolar lavage fluid has been detected following oesophagectomy[58,59,60] and levels correlate with the development of acute lung injury (ALI)/ARDS.[61,62,63] Postoperatively, patients are at risk from overspill and soiling the lung with gastric contents. Ultimately there is a high incidence of increased pulmonary vascular permeability following oeso-phagectomy.[64,65] This has encouraged some to practise fluid restriction and use mainly colloid infusions to try and limit extravascular lung water. Fluid restriction risks reducing cardiac output and should be monitored carefully. There is no evidence from randomised controlled trials that resuscitation with colloids in patients following surgery reduces the risk of death com-pared to resuscitation with crystalloids.[66] A recent study by Verheij and colleagues[67] examined the effects of fluid loading with crystalloid or colloid on the pulmonary leak index (PLI) and extravascular lung water in patients after cardiopulmonary bypass or vascular surgery. Both these types of opera-tions are also associated with a high incidence of ALI and 60% of their patients had high PLI at the start of the study protocol. They found that, providing fluid overload is avoided, the type of fluid used does not affect pulmonary permeability or oedema, except that HES (hydroxyethyl starch) 6% may ameliorate increased pulmonary permeability. It may be that the PiCCO® continuous cardiac output monitor that can measure extravascular lung water may be a valuable monitor. Ventilation strategies during one-lung ventilation may limit lung damage. There is evidence that limiting tidal volume,[68,69] pressure-controlled ventilation[70] and the application of the correct amount of positive end expiratory pressure (PEEP)[71,72,73,74] to the dependant lung may reduce lung injury and improve oxygenation. The correct amount of PEEP is not easy to determine. During one-lung ventilation there is an increase in intrinsic or auto PEEP and this varies between patients.[75] Inomata and colleagues[72] in a small study of eight patients identified that during one-lung ventilation when applied PEEP equalled intrinsic PEEP, oxygenation and oxygen delivery were highest and intrapulmonary shunting was minimised. Slinger and colleagues[73] applied PEEP of 5 cm H_2O during one-lung ventilation, studied its effects on oxygenation and related this to the static compliance curve. They found that if applied PEEP moved the final end-expiratory pressure nearer to the inflection point of the static compliance curve, which is the lung volume where the lungs change from poorly compliant to compliant, then oxygenation was improved. If applied PEEP moved the end-expiratory pressure further away from that inflection point, oxygenation was unaltered or worsened. Those with good lung function, i.e. with high FEV1 and little intrinsic PEEP to maintain lung volume in the dependant lung, were more likely to benefit from applied PEEP, but only six out of 42 patients had their PaO_2 improved by more than 20%. However, in this study during one-lung ventilation patients were ventilated with 100% oxygen, which may make a 20% improvement difficult to achieve. Valenza and colleagues[74] using static compliance tests confirmed that those with compliant lungs have the greatest decrease in compliance in the lateral position during one-lung ventilation and the application of PEEP in this group, ventilated with an inspired oxygen concentration to achieve a normal PaO_2, resulted in a 30% increase in oxygenation overall from a mean of 11.6 kPa to 15.3 kPa. In clinical practice, static compliance tests are not practical but many anaesthetists do now monitor dynamic compliance. The application of PEEP during one-lung ventilation improves compliance in some patients and affects it little in others. In Fig. 2.2, a dynamic compliance curve during one-lung volume-controlled ventilation, the application of PEEP moved the end expiratory pressure nearer to the inflection point, reduced peak airway pressure and markedly improved compliance.

Continuous positive airway pressure (CPAP) to the non-dependant lung will improve oxygenation[76] and theoretically limit the ischaemia/reperfusion injury. In practice the amount of CPAP to keep the lung expanded varies with lung compliance where the compliant lungs will remain inflated with very little CPAP. However, CPAP can interfere with surgical access. It is best to let the lung deflate to a small volume before applying CPAP and to keep it minimally inflated. Although inevitably retraction on the lung will

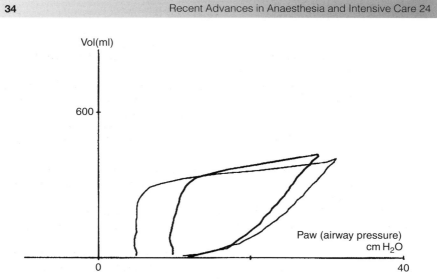

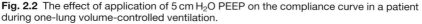

Fig. 2.2 The effect of application of 5 cm H_2O PEEP on the compliance curve in a patient during one-lung volume-controlled ventilation.

cause it to collapse further and it may need to be intermittently reinflated to maintain oxygenation.

Postoperative care

Historically patients were nursed postoperatively in an intensive care unit and received intermittent positive pressure ventilation overnight.[77] However, the increased use of epidural analgesia with short-acting anaesthetic drugs has encouraged a practice of early tracheal extubation and transfer to a high-dependency environment.[78,79,80] This has caused some debate but it is probably more important that there is careful patient selection and that high-risk patients are identified for level-3 care and goal-directed treatment. Following oesophagectomy all patients need to be managed by a team, including intensive care physicians, nurses and physiotherapists who have experience of managing these patients and are prompt and active in the detection and treatment of complications.

References

1. Sakata K, Hoshiyama Y, Morioka S, *et al*. JACC study group. Smoking, alcohol drinking and esophageal cancer: findings from the JACC study. *J Epidemiol* 2005; **15** (Suppl. 2): S212–19.
2. Lindblad M, Rodriguez LA, Lagergren J. Body mass, tobacco and alcohol and risk of esophageal, gastric cardia and gastric non-cardia adenocarcinoma among men and women in a nested case-control study. *Cancer Causes Control* 2005; **16**: 285–94.

3. Mortality and incidence trends for adenocarcinoma of the oesophagus in Queensland, 1982 to 2001. *Queensland Government Health Information Centre, Information Circular 66*, May 2004.

4. Jansson C, Johansson AL, Nyren O, Lagergren J. Socioeconomic factors and risk of esophageal adenocarcinoma: a nationwide Swedish case-control study. *Cancer Epidemiol Biomarkers Prev* 2005; **14**: 1754–61.

5. Allum WH, Griffin SM, Watson A, Colin-Jones D. Guidelines for the management of oesophageal and gastric cancer. *Gut* 2002; **50**(Suppl. V): 1–23.

6. Dimick JB, Wainess RM, Upchurch GR Jr., Iannettoni MD, Orringer MB. National trends in outcomes for esophageal resection. *Annals Thorac Surg* 2005; **79**: 212–16.

7. Kuo EY, Chang Y, Wright CD. Impact of hospital volume on clinical and economic outcomes for esophagectomy. *Ann Thorac Surg* 2001; **72**: 1118–24.

8. Swisher SG, DeFord L, Merriman KW, *et al.* Effect of operative volume on morbidity, mortality, and hospital use after esophagectomy for cancer. *J Thorac Cardiovasc Surg* 2000; **119**: 1126–32.

9. Patti MG, Corvera CU, Glasgow RE, Way LW. A hospital's annual rate of esophagectomy influences the operative mortality rate. *J Gastrointest Surg* 1998; **2**: 186–92.

10. Metzger R, Bollschweiler E, Vallbohmer D, *et al.* High-volume centers for esophagectomy: What is the number needed to achieve low postoperative mortality? *Dis Esophagus* 2004; **17**: 310–14.

11. Branagan G, Davis N. Early impact of centralization of oesophageal cancer surgery services. *Br J Surg* 2004; **91**: 1030–2.

12. Mariette C, Taillier G, Van Seuningen I, Triboulet JP. Factors affecting post-operative course and survival after en bloc resection for esophageal carcinoma. *Ann Thorac Surg* 2004; **78**: 1177–83.

13. Sutton DN, Wayman J, Griffin SM. Learning curve for oesophageal cancer surgery. *Br J Surg* 1998; **85**: 1399–402.

14. Matthews HR, Powell DJ, McConkey CC. Effects of surgical experience on the results of resection for oesophageal carcinoma. *Br J Surg* 1986; **73**: 621–3.

15. Anderson KB, Olsen JB, Pedersen JJ. Esophageal resections in Denmark. 1985–1988: A retrospective study of complications and early mortality. *Ugeskr Laeger* 1994; **156**: 473–6.

16. Miller JD, Jain MK, De Gara CJ, Morgan D, Urschel JD. Effect of surgical experience on results of esophagectomy for esophageal carcinoma. *J Surg Oncol* 1997; **65**: 20–1.

17. Aziz F, Khalil A, Hall JC. Evolution of trends in risk management. *ANZ J Surg* 2005; **75**: 603–7.

18. Rindani R, Martin CJ, Cox MR. Transhiatal versus Ivor – Lewis oesopha-gectomy: is there a difference? *ANZ J Surg* 1999; **69**: 187–94.

19. Kuwano H, Sumiyoshi K, Sonoda K, *et al.* Relationship between preoperative assessment of organ function and postoperative morbidity in patients with oesophageal cancer. *Eur J Surg* 1998; **164**: 581–6.

20. Bartels H, Stein HJ, Siewert JR. Preoperative risk analysis and postoperative mortality of oesophagectomy for resectable oesophageal cancer. *Br J Surg* 1998; **85**: 840–4.

21. Abunasra H, Lewis S, Beggs L, *et al*. Predictors of operative death after oesophagectomy for carcinoma. *Br J Surg* 2005; **92**: 1029–33.
22. Furguson MK, Durkin AE. Preoperative prediction of the risk of pulmonary complications after esophagectomy for cancer. *J Thorac Cardiovasc Surg* 2002; **123**: 661–9.
23. Bailey SH, Bull DA, Harpole DH, *et al*. Outcomes after oesophagectomy: a ten-year prospective cohort. *Ann Thorac Surg* 2003; **75**: 217–22.
24. Lin FC, Durkin AE, Ferguson MK. Induction therapy does not increase surgical morbidity after esophagectomy for cancer. *Ann Thorac Surg* 2004; **78**: 1783–9.
25. Nagawa H, Kobori O, Muto T. Prediction of pulmonary complications after transthoracic oesophagectomy. *Br J Surg* 1994; **81**: 860–2.
26. Tandon S, Batchelor A, Bullock R, *et al*. Peri-operative risk factors for acute lung injury after elective oesophagectomy. *Br J Anaesth* 2001; **86**: 633–8.
27. Law S, Wong K-H, Kwok K-F, Chu K-M, Wong J. Predictive factors for postoperative pulmonary complications and mortality after esophagectomy for cancer. *Ann Surg* 2004; **240**: 791–800.
28. Ferguson MK, Martin TR, Reeder KB, Olak J. Mortality after esophagectomy: risk-factor analysis. *World J Surg* 1997; **21**: 599–603.
29. Atkins BZ, Shah AS, Hutcheson KA, *et al*. Reducing hospital morbidity and mortality following esophagectomy. *Ann Thorac Surg* 2004; **78**: 1170–6.
30. Noze T, Kinura Y, Ishida M, *et al*. Correlation of pre-operative nutritional condition with post-operative complications in surgical treatment for oeso-phageal carcinoma. *Eur J Surg Oncol* 2002; **28**: 396–400.
31. Fiorica F, Di Bona D, Schepis F, *et al*. Preoperative chemoradiotherapy for oesophageal cancer: a systemic review and meta-analysis. *Gut* 2004; **53**: 925–30.
32. Imdahl A, Schoffel U, Ruf G. Impact of neoadjuvant therapy on perioperative morbidity in patients with oesophageal cancer. *Am J Surg* 2004; **187**: 64–8.
33. Abou–Jawde RM, Mekhail T, Adelstein DJ, *et al*. Impact of induction con-current chemoradiotherapy on pulmonary function and postoperative acute respiratory complications in esophageal cancer. *Chest* 2005; **128**: 250–5.
34. Eguchi R, Ide H, Nakamura T, *et al*. Analysis of postoperative complications after esophagectomy for oesophageal cancer in patients receiving neoadjuvant therapy. *Jpn J Thor Cardiovasc Surg* 1999; **47**: 552–8.
35. Liedman B, Johnsson E, Merke C, Ruth M, Lundell L. Preoperative adjuvant radiochemotherapy may increase the risk in patients undergoing thoracoab-dominal esophageal resections. *Dig Surg* 2001; **18**: 169–75.
36. Groves J, Edwards ND, Carr B, Sherry KM. Perioperative myocardial ischae-mia, heart rate and arrhythmia in patients undergoing thoracotomy: an observational study. *Br J Anaesth* 1999; **83**: 850–4.
37. Older P, Hall A, Hader R. Cardiopulmonary exercise testing as a screening test for perioperative management of major surgery in the elderly. *Chest* 1999; **116**: 355–62.
38. Zafirellis KD, Fountoulakis A, Dolan K, *et al*. Evaluation of POSSUM in patients with oesophageal cancer undergoing resection. *Br J Surg* 2002; **89**: 1150–5.
39. McCulloch P, Ward J, Tekkis PP, for the ASCOT group of surgeons, on behalf of the British Oesophago-Gastric Cancer Group. Mortality and morbidity in gastro-oesophageal cancer surgery: initial results of ASCOT multicentre pro-spective cohort study. *BMJ* 2003; **327**: 1192–7.

40. Tekkis PP, McCulloch P, Poloniecki JD, *et al.* Risk-adjusted prediction of operative mortality in oesophagogastric surgery with O-POSSUM. *Br J Surg* 2004; **91**: 288–95.

41. Gocmen E, Koc M, Tez M, *et al.* Evaluation of P-POSSUM and O-POSSUM scores in patients with gastric cancer undergoing resection. *Hepato-Gastroenterology* 2004; **51**: 1864–6.

42. Hlatky MA, Boineau RE, Higginbotham MB, *et al.* A brief self-administered questionnaire to determine functional capacity (the Duke Activity Status Index). *Am J Cardiol* 1989; **64**: 651–4.

43. Nagamatsu Y, Shima I, Yamana H, *et al.* Preoperative evaluation of cardio-pulmonary reserve with the use of expired gas analysis during exercise testing in patients with squamous cell carcinoma of the thoracic esophagus. *J Thorac Cardiovasc Surg* 2001; **121**: 1064–8.

44. Murthy SC, Law S, Whooley BP, *et al.* Atrial fibrillation after esophagectomy is a marker for postoperative morbidity and mortality. *J Thorac Cardiovasc Surg* 2003; **126**: 1162–7.

45. Boyd O, Grounds RM, Bennett ED. A randomised clinical trial of the effect of deliberate perioperative increase of oxygen delivery on mortality in high-risk surgical patients. *JAMA* 1993; **270**: 2699–707.

46. Wilson J, Woods I, Fawcett J, *et al.* Reducing the risk of major elective surgery: randomised controlled trial of preoperative optimisation of oxygen delivery. *BMJ* 1999; **318**: 1099–103.

47. Boyd O, Lamb G, Mackay CJ, Grounds RM, Bennett ED. A comparison of the efficacy of dopexamine and dobutamine for increasing oxygen delivery in high-risk surgical patients. *Anaesth Intensive Care* 1995; **23**: 478–84.

48. Renton MC, Snowden CP. Dopexamine and its role in the protection of hepatosplanchnic and renal perfusion in high-risk surgical and critically ill patients. *Br J Anaesth* 2005; **94**: 459–67.

49. Oberbeck R, Schmitz D, Schuler M, *et al.* Dopexamine and cellular immune functions during systemic inflammation. *Immunobiology* 2004; **208**: 429–38.

50. Kusano C, Baba M, Takao S, *et al.* Oxygen delivery as a factor in the development of fatal postoperative complications after oesophagectomy. *Br J Surg* 1997; **84**: 252–7.

51. Block BM, Liu SS, Rowlingson A J, *et al.* Efficacy of postoperative epidural analgesia: a meta-analysis. *JAMA* 2003; **290**: 2455–63.

52. Rodgers A, Walker N, Schug S, *et al.* Reduction in postoperative mortality and morbidity with epidural or spinal anaesthesia: results from overview of randomized trials. *BMJ* 2000; **321**: 1493–7.

53. Liberi S, Markou N, Sakayianni K, *et al.* Coronary artery disease and upper abdominal surgery; impact of anesthesia on perioperative myocardial ischaemia. *Hepato-Gastroenterol* 2003; **50**: 1814–20.

54. Yeager MP, Glass DD, Neff RK, Brink-Johnsen T. Epidural anesthesia and analgesia in high-risk surgical patients. *Anesthesiology* 1987; **66**: 729–36.

55. Kehlet H, Holte K. Review of postoperative ileus. *Am J Surg* 2001; **182**(5A Suppl.): S3–10.

56. Crozier TA, Sydow M, Siewert JR, Braun U. Postoperative pulmonary complication rate and long-term changes in respiratory function following eso-phagectomy with esophagogastrostomy. *Acta Anaesthesiol Scand* 1992; **36**: 10–5.

57. Jordan S, Mitchell JA, Quinlan GJ, Goldstraw P, Evans T W. The pathogenesis of lung injury following pulmonary resection. *Eur Resp J* 2000; **15**: 790–9.

58. Sato N, Koeda K, Kimura Y, *et al.* Cytokine profile of serum and broncho-alveolar lavage fluids following thoracic esophageal cancer surgery. *Eur Surg Res* 2001; **33**: 279–84.

59. Cree RTJ, Warnell I, Staunton M, Shaw I, *et al.* Alveolar and plasma concentrations of interleukin-8 and vascular endothelial growth factor following oesophagectomy. *Anaesthesia* 2004; **59**: 867–71.

60. Nakanishi K, Takeda S, Terajima K, Takano T, Ogawa R. Myocardial dysfunction associated with proinflammatory cytokines after esophageal resection. *Anesth Analg* 2000; **91**: 270–5.

61. Schilling MK, Gassmann N, Sigurdsson GH, *et al.* Role of thromboxane and leukotriene B4 in patients with acute respiratory distress syndrome after oesophagectomy. *Br J Anaesth* 1998; **80**: 36–40.

62. Kooguchi K, Kobayashi A, Kitamura Y, *et al.* Elevated expression of inducible nitric oxide synthase and inflammatory cytokines in the alveolar macrophages after esophagectomy. *Crit Care Med* 2002; **30**: 71–6.

63. Katsuta T, Saito T, Shigemitsu Y, *et al.* Relation between tumour necrosis factor alpha and interleukin 1 beta producing capacity of peripheral monocytes and pulmonary complications following oesophagectomy. *Br J Surg* 1998; **85**: 548–53.

64. Reid PT, Donnelly SC, MacGregor IR, *et al.* Pulmonary endothelial permeability and circulating neutrophil–endothelial markers in patients undergoing esophagogastrectomy. *Crit Care Med* 2000; **28**: 3161–5.

65. Baudouin SV. Lung injury after thoracotomy. *Br J Anaesth* 2003; **91**: 132–42.

66. Roberts I, Alderson P, Bunn F, *et al.* Colloids versus crystalloids for fluid resuscitation in critically ill patients. *The Cochrane Database of Systematic Reviews* 2004, Issue 4. Art. No: CD000567.

67. Verheij J, van Lingen A, Raijmakers PGHM, *et al.* Effect of fluid loading with saline or colloids on pulmonary permeability, oedema and lung injury score after cardiac and major vascular surgery. *Br J Anaesth* 2006; **96**: 21–30.

68. Schilling T, Kozian A, Huth C, *et al.* The pulmonary immune effects of mechanical ventilation in patients undergoing thoracic surgery. *Anesth Analg* 2005; **101**: 957–65.

69. The Acute Respiratory Distress Syndrome Network. Ventilation with lower tidal volumes as compared with traditional tidal volumes for acute lung injury and the acute respiratory distress syndrome. *N Engl J Med* 2000; **342**: 1301–8.

70. Turul M, Camci E, Karadeniz H, Senturk M, Pembeci K, Akpir K. Comparison of volume controlled with pressure controlled ventilation during one-lung anaesthesia. *Br J Anaesth* 1997; **79**: 306–10.

71. Senturk NM, Dilek A, Camci E, *et al.* Effects of positive end-expiratory pressure on ventilatory and oxygenation parameters during pressure-controlled one-lung ventilation. *J Cardiothorac Vasc Anesth* 2005; **19**: 71–5.

72. Inomata S, Nishikawa T, Saito S, Kihara S. "Best" PEEP during one-lung ventilation. *Br J Anaesth* 1997; **78**: 754–6.

73. Slinger PD, Kruger M, McRae K, Winton T. Relation of the static compliance curve and positive end-expiratory pressure to oxygenation during one-lung ventilation. *Anesthesiology* 2001; **95**: 1096–102.

74. Valenza F, Ronzoni G, Perrone L, *et al.* Positive end-expiratory pressure applied to the dependant lung during one-lung ventilation improves oxygenation and respiratory mechanics in patients with high FEV_1. *Eur J Anaesthesiol* 2004; **21**: 938–43.

75. Slinger PD, Hickey DR. The interaction between applied PEEP and auto-PEEP during one-lung ventilation. *J Cardiothorac Vasc Anesth* 1998; **12**: 133–6.
76. Slinger P, Triolet W, Wilson J. Improving arterial oxygenation during one-lung ventilation. *Anesthesiology* 1988; **68**: 291–5.
77. Shah M, Pearce A. Oesophagectomy and elective postoperative ventilation. *Br J Anaesth* 2004; **92**: 907–8.
78. Ghosh S, Steyn RS, Marzouk JF, *et al.* The effectiveness of high-dependency units in the management of high-risk thoracic surgical cases. *Eur J Cardiothorac Surg* 2004; **25**: 123–6.
79. Chandrashekar MV, Irving M, Wayman J, Raimes SA, Linsley A. Immediate extubation and epidural analgesia allow safe management in a high-dependency unit after two-stage oesophagectomy. Results of eight years of experience in a specialized upper gastrointestinal unit in a district general hospital. *Br J Anaesth* 2003; **90**: 474–9.
80. Rocker M, Havard TJ, Wagle A. Early extubation after two-stage oesophagectomy. *Br J Anaesth* 2003; **91**: 760.

CHAPTER 3

Matt M. Thompson and Ian Loftus

Vascular surgery

In the last five years, vascular surgery has undergone a considerable change in emphasis with respect to the breadth of conditions being treated and in the techniques used in therapy. The evidence base for vascular surgical intervention has broadened considerably, particularly in the fields of carotid intervention and the treatment of abdominal and thoracic aortic aneurysms. This newly gathered evidence base has been used to further define the indications for vascular reconstruction.

The emphasis on the development of new techniques for vascular intervention has continued, with the focus on minimally invasive and endovascular therapy. The application of endovascular therapy for the treatment of aortic and carotid disease is still largely confined to specialist centres but these techniques are likely to represent the future of vascular intervention. The change in direction of traditional vascular surgery has significant implications for anaesthetic practice as most of the newer vascular techniques are amenable to loco-regional anaesthesia. This chapter reviews the most recent advances in vascular practice for the treatment of aortic disease, carotid artery stenosis and varicose veins.

Advances in the treatment of abdominal aortic aneurysms

Aortic aneurysms are responsible for 13 000 deaths in the UK, with abdominal aneurysms causing 8000 of these.[1] The principles that guide aneurysm treatment are to detect aneurysms prior to rupture, to electively repair these aneurysms with the lowest possible mortality and to treat the complications of aneurysmal disease (primarily rupture). Unfortunately,

Recent Advances in Anaesthesia and Intensive Care 24, ed. J. N. Cashman and R. M. Grounds.
Published by Cambridge University Press. © Cambridge University Press 2007.

the majority of aneurysms are asymptomatic and many rupture before elective surgical repair can be contemplated. The community mortality of ruptured abdominal aortic aneurysms (AAA) exceeds 80%.

In recent years, significant progress has been made in the early detection of AAA with the adoption of screening programmes and in reducing surgical mortality with the introduction of endovascular repair of abdominal aneurysms.

Screening programmes

Community-based screening programmes aim to identify AAA in a population with a significant prevalence of the disease (elderly males), who would benefit from elective repair. Most screening programmes have reported a 4–5% prevalence of AAA in males over 60 years of age, and there have been reports that community-screening programmes can reduce mortality from ruptured AAA. Community-based screening has recently been subjected to a rigorous multicentre randomised controlled clinical trial.

In the Multicentre Aneurysm Screening Study (MASS),[2] 67 800 males aged 65–74 years were randomised to invitation-based community screening or no screening. Eighty percent of the invited group accepted the offer of screening and this group demonstrated a 53% reduction in death from aneurysm rupture. The cost effectiveness was £8000 per life year gained at ten years follow up, which compares favourably with other nationally accepted programmes. These data suggested that screening programmes for AAA should be instituted, and discussions are at an advanced stage in the UK. Adoption of an aneurysm screening programme would have significant implication for workload, with a marked rise in the number of elective aneurysms being treated and a reduction in ruptured aneurysm surgery. It has been estimated that for a population of 350 000, a screening programme would lead to two additional elective AAA operations per month, and save 11 AAA-related deaths per year.[3]

Endovascular aneurysm repair

Endovascular aneurysm repair involves the exclusion of an aneurysm from the circulation using a stent-graft that is delivered to the aneurysm via the femoral arteries (Fig. 3.1 a, b, c). Most endovascular grafts are designed as a modular reconstruction which is assembled within the aneurysm sac (Fig. 3.2). Standard endovascular aneurysm repair can only be performed if there is an adequate fixation zone between the renal arteries and the start of the aneurysm to allow adequate anchorage of the stent.

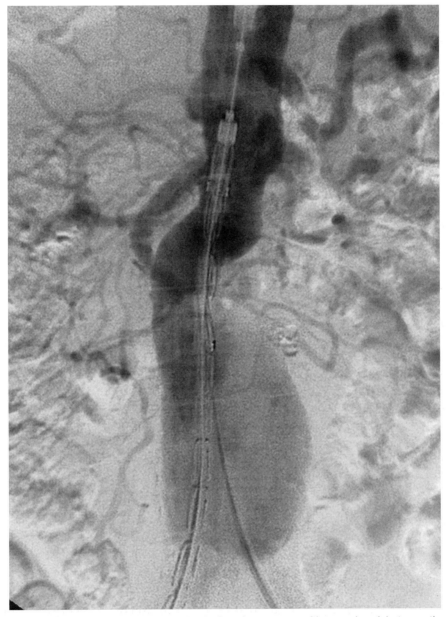

Fig. 3.1a Angiogram illustrating an abdominal aortic aneurysm with a good neck between the renal arteries and the aneurysm. An endovascular stent-graft within the delivery sheath has been introduced through the aneurysm.

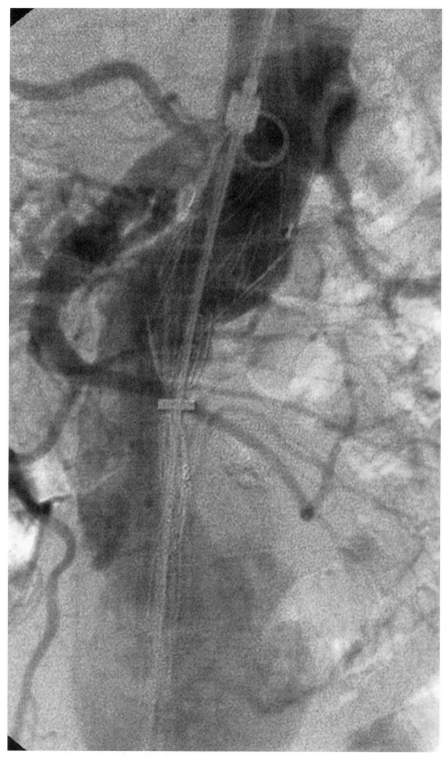

Fig. 3.1b The endovascular graft has been partially deployed at the level of the renal arteries.

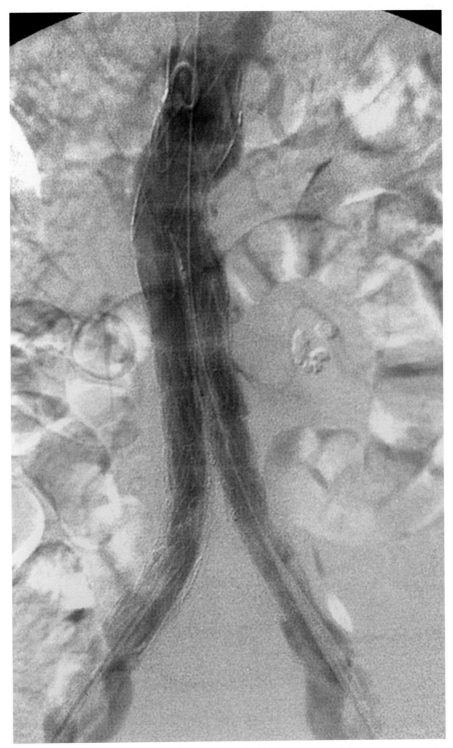

Fig. 3.1c The completed endovascular repair. The modular graft has been completely deployed to exclude the aneurysm from the circulation.

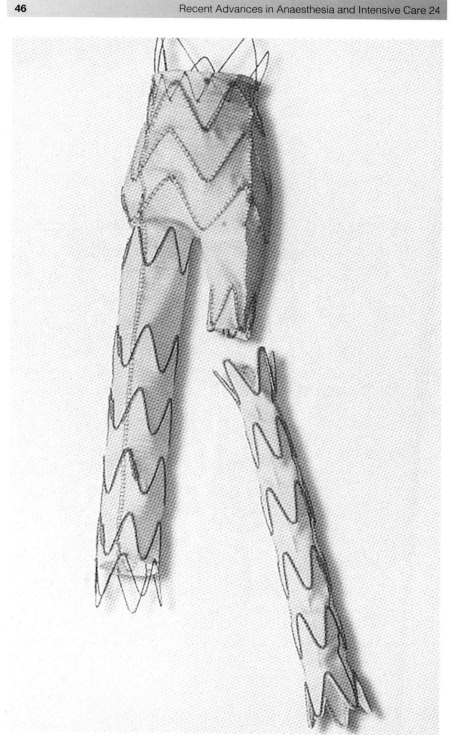

Fig. 3.2 A modular bifurcated endovascular stent-graft.

Most series report that 50–70% of AAA are anatomically suitable for endovascular repair.[4]

The potential advantages of endovascular aneurysm repair relate to the minimally invasive nature of the procedure, with both a laparotomy and aortic cross-clamping being avoided. The reduction in operative extent leads to a reduction in physiological stress with cardiac, respiratory, metabolic and renal parameters being improved in comparison to conventional surgical procedures.[5,6,7] It was hoped that the reduction in physiological stress associated with endovascular repair would translate to a reduction in the mortality and morbidity of elective aneurysm repair. In most consecutive series and registries this promise appeared to hold true with conventional aneurysm repair having a mortality of 7%[8] as compared to 1–3% for endovascular procedures.[9] In addition, endovascular aneurysm repair was promoted as a technique that could be used safely in patients who were unfit for conventional surgery.[10]

Despite the mortality advantages, endovascular aneurysm repair did not find universal acceptance as there were some doubts surrounding the durability of the procedure, with some patients developing a leak between the aortic stent and the aneurysm wall ('endoleak'; Fig. 3.3) that predisposed to aneurysm rupture.[11] Other concerns over durability included a small but definite incidence of stent fracture, graft fatigue and migration of the endograft.

The debate over the place of endovascular repair has recently been clarified by a series of randomised controlled trials[12,13,14,15,16] that have compared endovascular and conventional surgery in patients fit for conventional procedures, and compared endovascular repair against best medical therapy in patients unfit for conventional surgery. The headline findings of the EVAR 1 trial (endovascular vs. conventional surgery in fit patients) are illustrated in Table 3.1. Endovascular repair was associated with a threefold reduction in operative mortality, a long-term decrease in aneurysm-related mortality, and an increase in cost. The trial demonstrated no difference in overall mortality at four years in the two groups, but it is questionable whether the trial was adequately powered to investigate this end point. The EVAR 1 trial also demonstrated an increased reintervention rate in the endovascular group, but this did not appear to be associated with any additional mortality.

Together with previous studies, the trials have suggested that endovascular repair is the safest option in fit patients with anatomy suitable for endovascular repair. The recent NCEPOD report (Abdominal Aortic

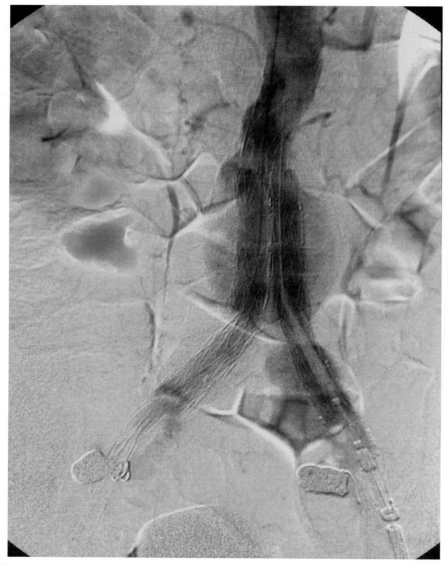

Fig. 3.3 Endovascular aneurysm repair demonstrating a leak between the stent and the aortic wall. The leak results in contrast filling the aneurysm sac. If left untreated, this endoleak would predispose to aneurysm rupture.

Aneurysms – A Service In Need of Surgery; www.ncepod.org.uk/2005report2/ Downloads/AAA%20Surgical%20Questionniare.pdf) summarised that 'endovascular repair is significantly more efficacious in preventing aneurysm-related death than operative repair and should be offered to all patients in this category (fit for open repair)'. There are still issues to be resolved regarding the long-term durability in young patients, but a

Table 3.1 Table illustrating the main results of the EVAR 1 trial which randomised fit patients to either open or endovascular aneurysm repair.

	EVAR	Open repair
In hospital mortality (intention to treat)	2.1%	6.2%
In hospital mortality (per protocol)	1.6%	6.0%
Aneurysm-related mortality (4 year)	4%	7%
All-cause mortality (4 year)	26%	29%
Cost (4 year)	£13258	£9945

significant increase in the number of endovascular repairs should be expected in forthcoming years.

In contrast to the encouraging results in the EVAR 1 trial, the results of EVAR 2 were unexpected. The EVAR 2 randomised patients unfit for conventional surgery, to endovascular repair or best medical therapy. The results demonstrated that the perioperative mortality for the endovascular group was 9% and that there was no difference in overall mortality between the two groups after four year follow up. The conclusions from these results were that endovascular repair of aneurysms in unfit patients did not offer any survival benefit and that, in these patients, consideration should be given to improving fitness prior to treatment of the aneurysm.

Anaesthetic implications of endovascular aneurysm repair

The results of the recent trials suggest that endovascular aneurysm repair will assume a greater importance in the management of infra-renal aneurysms. This may have significant implications for the mode of anaesthesia employed for these patients. Both local and regional anaesthetic techniques have been utilised in patients undergoing endovascular aneurysm repair. Most trials to date have demonstrated no difference in mortality or morbidity rates between different forms of anaesthesia,[17,18] but one recent non-randomised study has suggested lower mortality with local anaesthesia.[19]

Endovascular repair of ruptured AAA

The operative mortality for open repair of ruptured AAA has remained high (40–50%) for the last decade. The mortality may be related to the physiological consequence of laparotomy and aortic clamping in patients who have already suffered massive blood loss. Endovascular repair has been advocated as an attractive solution to ruptured aneurysm surgery owing to the lesser physiological stress of the procedure. Several units have demonstrated that endovascular repair of ruptured aneurysms presents a considerable logistical challenge, but that in experienced centres it is an attractive option to conventional surgery.[20]

At present, the evidence base for endovascular repair of ruptured aneurysms is not impressive, but single-centre series have shown encouraging results. The one randomised trial performed so far revealed similar mortality for open or endovascular repair. However, it remains likely that endovascular surgery will assume a greater role in repair of ruptured aneurysms in the next decade.

Advances in the treatment of thoracic and thoracoabdominal aortic disease

The treatment of thoracic and thoracoabdominal aortic disease provides one of the biggest challenges in cardiovascular practice. The range of conditions is vast and includes aortic aneurysms, aortic dissections, traumatic aortic transactions, penetrating aortic ulcers, intramural haematomas and mycotic aneurysms. The traditional surgical approach has been to replace the diseased segment of aorta with a prosthetic graft, usually through a left-sided thoracotomy. To achieve good results several adjunctive procedures are required to maintain perfusion of the viscera and spinal cord.[21,22] These manoeuvres include distal aortic perfusion through left heart bypass, selective visceral and intercostal perfusion, CSF drainage, intercostal re-implantation and epidural cooling. Despite these efforts the results of open surgery on the thoracic aorta remain poor, with registries reporting a 30% mortality rate at one year.[23] A recent report (2001) from the Society of Cardiothoracic Surgeons of Great Britain and Ireland (www.scts.org) revealed a 31% mortality rate for replacement of the descending thoracic aorta.

Endovascular surgery of the thoracic aorta

Endovascular surgery of the thoracic aorta followed the development of endovascular techniques for the abdominal aorta, and utilises the same principles. The thoracic aorta may be treated with a straight endovascular prosthesis introduced through the femoral artery. The graft is anchored proximally in the proximal descending thoracic aorta or the distal aortic arch; and distally in the thoracic aorta above the coeliac axis. The attraction of this technique is that graft placement is relatively straightforward and it avoids the thoracotomy, and visceral and spinal ischaemia that complicates open repair.

Endovascular repair for thoracic aortic pathology has been introduced rapidly into widespread clinical practice as early results have demonstrated

Table 3.2 Table illustrating the main results from a concurrent cohort trial of open and endovascular repair of descending thoracic aneurysms.

	Endovascular repair	Open repair
30-day mortality	2.1%	11.7%
30-day paraplegia	3%	14%
30-day stroke	4%	4%
Freedom from major adverse events (3 year)	58%	20%

significant advantages over conventional surgical techniques, with an improvement in elective mortality of between 10–20%. The Eurostar registry of 200 procedures reported an elective mortality of 5.3% for thoracic aneurysms and 6% for the treatment of Type B thoracic aortic dissections. In this series the paraplegia rate was 4%, which compares very favourably with the 10% reported in many open surgical series.[24] Similarly, Sayed and Thompson performed a meta-analysis of thoracic aortic procedures in 2005. This analysis demonstrated a 30-day mortality of 4% for thoracic aneurysms, 8% for dissections and 8% for traumatic ruptures. The overall paraplegia rate was 1.3% and stroke rate 1.7%.[25]

Owing to the initial experiences reported for thoracic endografting, there have been no randomised trials performed, as it has been argued that the mortality rates between the endovascular and open procedures are too disparate to make randomisation possible. There has been one concurrent cohort study published which has demonstrated the superiority of endovascular thoracic aneurysm repair over a concurrent series of open surgical procedures. The results of this trial are summarised in Table 3.2.[26,27]

In the United Kingdom the National Institute for Health and Clinical Excellence (NICE) has recently issued guidelines on thoracic endografting. The guidance suggests that endovascular repair of the thoracic aorta is a suitable alternative to conventional surgery provided that appropriate protocols and arrangements for governance are in place. The guidelines also suggest that the procedure should be performed by a multidisciplinary team and that facilities for cardiothoracic surgery and cardiopulmonary bypass should be in place. Given the very significant differences in operative mortality between open and endovascular surgery, it is likely that most descending thoracic pathology will be treated by endovascular procedures in the near future.

The indications for these procedures may be expanded to include arch aneurysms by transposition and bypass of the great vessels, which allows the graft to be anchored across the aortic arch (Fig. 3.4 a, b).

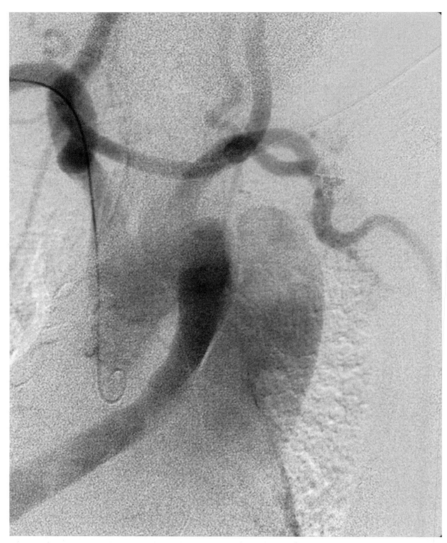

Fig. 3.4 a, b Endovascular repair of a chronic dissection with aneurysmal expansion. The pre-operative angiogram (a) demonstrates a carotid–carotid bypass. Following deployment of the endovascular graft (b) the aneurysm has been excluded.

Hybrid and fenestrated procedures for thoracoabdominal aneurysms

The expansion in endovascular techniques has been applied to the treatment of thoracoabdominal aneurysms. These aneurysms are difficult to treat with conventional techniques and have historically been associated with the worst outcomes, often owing to the involvement of the visceral and renal vessels in the aneurysmal process. In recent months, a hybrid approach has been described to treat these lesions. This approach combines bypasses to the

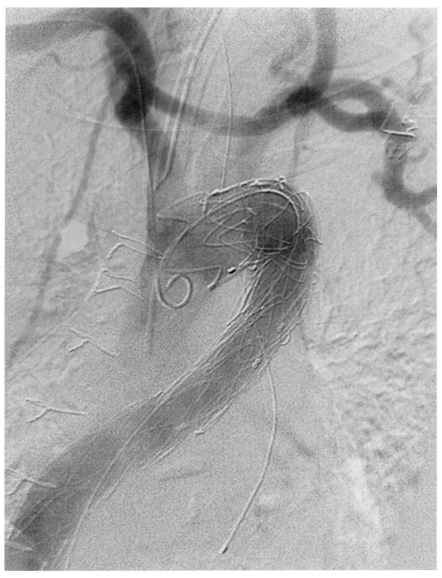

Fig. 3.4 a, b (cont.)

visceral and renal vessels, with endovascular repair of the entire thoracoab-dominal aorta (Fig. 3.5 a, b). Early results of this approach are promising, but are likely to remain in specialist centres for the time being.

An alternative technique is to use an endovascular graft with custom-made fenestrations and branches for the visceral vessels. These grafts are now

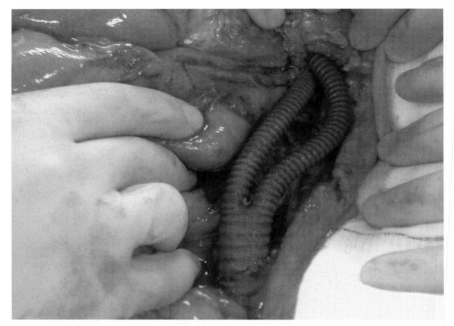

Fig. 3.5 Patient with a thoracoabdominal aneurysm: (a) a hybrid procedure has been performed with an iliac to superior mesenteric and coeliac bypass; (b) preceding endovascular repair.

being applied more widely[28]and are most suited for infra-renal aneurysms without an adequate proximal neck for fixation (Fig. 3.6).

Developments in carotid surgical practice

The role of carotid endarterectomy (CEA) in the management of sympto-matic carotid disease is well established.[29] The role of surgery in asympto-matic patients has been more controversial, though the two large randomised trials performed thus far have suggested a benefit from surgery in selected patients.[30,31] This benefit of CEA, particularly in asymptomatic patients, relies heavily on a low perioperative stroke and death rate. The adoption of CEA as the preferred treatment for patients with asymptomatic disease has not been universal, and the issue is now confounded by changes in what may be accepted as 'best medical therapy', and improvements in carotid stenting techniques.

Over the years, there has been much debate about many aspects of the surgical techniques used during CEA, and the relative contribution to peri-operative morbidity and mortality. It has been suggested that this may depend to an extent on the type of anaesthetic used.

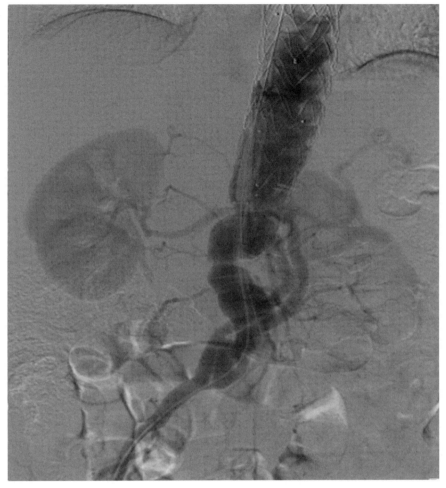

Fig. 3.5 (cont.)

The role of local anaesthesia for CEA

Local anaesthesia (LA) for CEA involves superficial and deep cervical plexus blockade supplemented by local infiltration. It has been used during CEA for the past four decades. The proponents of the technique suggest that it allows for the selective use of carotid shunts to maintain cerebral blood flow during arterial cross-clamping. There are certainly very occasional complications associated with the routine use of shunts, such as inadvertent, unrecognised occlusion or distal internal carotid dissection. Some surgeons argue, however, that under LA the patient has to lie still in an uncomfortable position for a long period of time and swallowing can make fine dissection and difficult reconstruction more complex and risky. Also, in the event of problems, urgent intubation is more difficult.

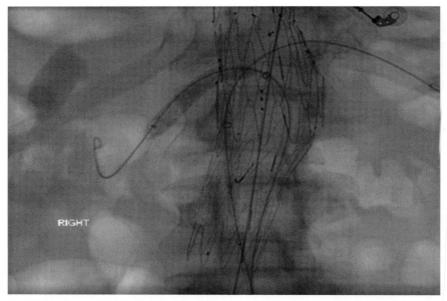

RIGHT

Fig. 3.6 Deployment of a fenestrated graft for a juxta-renal aneurysm. This graft has fenestrations for two renal stents.

The GALA trial (general anaesthetic versus local anaesthetic for carotid surgery) is currently underway in the UK. The GALA trial is a multicentre, randomised trial assessing the relative risks of cardiac events, stroke and death following CEA. It has recently randomised the 2000th patient.

There have been many non-randomised studies which suggest that CEA under LA is associated with a lower operative risk of stroke and death than CEA under general anaesthetic (GA). There have been a number of previous randomised trials, and a recent Cochrane review, which included 7 trials and 41 non-randomised studies, involving 25 622 operations.[32] Meta-analysis of the non-randomised trials revealed a significant reduction in the risk of death (35 studies), stroke (31 studies), stroke or death (26 studies), myocardial infarction (22 studies) and pulmonary complications (7 studies) within 30 days of the operation. Meta-analysis of the randomised trial data revealed a non-significant trend for LA towards reduced mortality within 30 days and post-operative haemorrhage but no difference in stroke rates. There is currently, however, insufficient evidence to recommend the routine use of LA in preference to GA, and the results of the randomised trial are awaited with interest.

The role of carotid stenting
The endovascular stent treatment of carotid disease is growing as an alternative to surgery, especially for patients at high operative risk. There are

limited trial data at present to directly support stenting in preference to CEA, though evidence from the major registries and large single-centre studies would support a possible role. Carotid stenting should currently be performed in centers with experience, with the use of cerebral protection devices.

The SAPPHIRE trial (Stenting and Angioplasty with Protection in Patients at High Risk for Endarterectomy) randomised 334 patients with co-existing conditions that potentially increased the risk posed by CEA, to CEA or stenting with embolus protection.[33] Criteria for inclusion were symptomatic stenosis > 50%, or asymptomatic stenosis > 80%. Of 747 patients enrolled, only 334 underwent randomisation for a variety of reasons. Subsequently, 151/167 underwent CEA and 159/167 were stented, of which 80% and 82% were asymptomatic respectively. Looking at the primary end point of death, stroke or myocardial infarction (MI) to 30 days, plus stroke/stroke related death to one year, there was a benefit from stenting that just reached significance for superiority (12.2% and 20.1% for stenting and CEA respectively). The fundamental point of this trial, however, was the very poor outcomes that were reported in asymptomatic patients. With the high stroke and death rates in this group of patients, very few would have derived any benefit from the procedure.

CAVATAS (Carotid and Vertebral Artery Transluminal Angioplasty Study) demonstrated no difference between stenting and CEA in 504 symptomatic patients, with a 30-day major stroke and death rate of 5.9% and 6.4% for stenting and surgery respectively.[34] There was no difference at one year or three years, the latter rates for any stroke and death documented as 14.3% for stent, and 14.2% for CEA.

The Lexington study of 104 symptomatic patients randomised to CEA or stent reported one early death in the surgery group, and one transient ischaemic attack in the stent group.[35] No further major events were described at two years for either group. Conversely, the Leicester study was stopped after randomisation of 17 patients after 5/7 in the stent group suffered a cerebrovascular accident (CVA).[36]

The other major trials currently under way will help to clarify the future role of carotid stenting. It may well be that there is a specific role for the treatment of carotid disease in high-risk surgical patients, or conversely for asymptomatic patients. It should be recognised that the practice is still evolving.

Developments in the treatment of varicose veins

Symptoms of varicose veins are extremely variable and many operations are performed for purely cosmetic indications. Minimally invasive techniques, which offer a better cosmetic result and potentially lower complication rates compared to conventional surgery, are therefore an attractive option. Furthermore, they enable immediate mobilisation and early return to work. There are concerns about recurrence rates and long-term studies are awaited with interest. Less invasive options include injection sclerotherapy, and endoluminal ablation techniques.

Injection sclerotherapy

Sclerotherapy involves direct injection of a chemical sclerosant, usually sodium tetradecyl sulphate (STD), into the vein, initiating thrombophlebitis and fibrosis. More recently, this has been performed under ultrasound guidance directly into the long or short saphenous vein (LSV/SSV). Foam sclerotherapy employs the same principles, performed using a smaller quantity of sclerosant such as polidocanol 0.5% which by agitation, pre-injection, turns to foam. A controlled clinical trial of liquid versus foam sclerotherapy to treat long saphenous incompetence, revealed much better success rates for foam.[37] In a further non-controlled trial, while the clinical recurrence rate was comparable to surgery (8% at one year), the duplex occlusion rate was only 67%.[38]

Some concerns have been raised about the potential for foam embolisation causing complications. The United States Food and Drug Administration halted a clinical phase-2 trial of a commercial preparation of polidocanol microfoam in 2003 because of concerns relating to possible gas embolism. Neurological complications such as transient visual disturbances and confusional states have also been reported. However, a large multicentre registry of over 12 000 sclerotherapy sessions reported no long-term neurological sequelae and only one deep vein thrombosis.[39]

Endovenous laser ablation

Laser therapy for varicose veins offers a true potential advantage that it can be performed under local anaesthetic in an outpatient setting.[40] The technique involves cannulation of the LSV or SSV under ultrasound guidance and a Seldinger technique to pass a narrow gauge sheath to the junction with the deep vein. An 810-nm diode laser fibre is positioned 2 cm from the junction (Fig. 3.7). Perivenous tumescent infiltration of 0.1% lignocaine is then performed, under ultrasound guidance, around the full length of the vein. This provides excellent analgesia but also compresses the vein onto the laser ensuring good apposition, and acts as a heat sink to prevent thermal damage to surrounding tissues, particularly nerves. The laser is

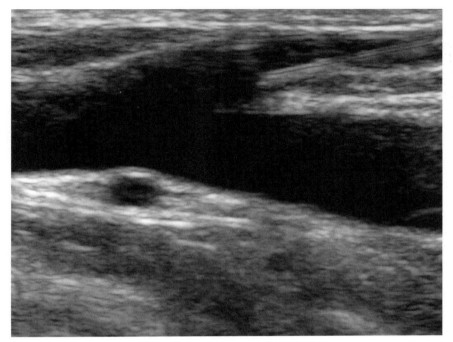

Fig. 3.7 Ultrasound image of an endovenous laser ablation. The laser tip is positioned just proximal to the sapheno-femoral junction.

fired as it is gradually withdrawn from the vein and on completion a compression bandage or stocking is applied.

The early results from laser therapy were promising, with successful application and tolerance. Side effects were very few, with most experiencing mild bruising and discomfort for one to two weeks. Longer-term results are even more promising. Concerns regarding possible recurrence rates seem ill founded. In a study of 499 veins treated in 423 patients over 3 years, successful closure was achieved in 490 after the initial treatment[41,42] and 113/121 (93.4%) remain closed at two years follow up on duplex ultrasound. There were no burns, long-term paraesthesia or deep vein thromboses reported. There have currently been no randomised trials reported in the literature. Laser therapy for varicose veins seems to be a very safe and effective treatment option with minor side effects, and data from clinical trials are eagerly awaited.

A minimally invasive approach to varicose vein treatment is popular with patients, for what is largely a cosmetic problem. Long-term results must be as good as, if not better than, conventional surgery. Low rates of complications are achievable, and early ambulation and return to work encouraged.

Further, there are cost implications, with new techniques cost effective rather than more expensive, with a shift away from inpatient to an out-patient-based practice.

References

1. Thompson MM. Infrarenal abdominal aortic aneurysms. *Curr Treat Options Cardiovasc Med* 2003; **5**: 137–46.
2. Ashton HA, Buxton MJ, Day NE, *et al.* The Multicentre Aneurysm Screening Study (MASS) into the effect of abdominal aortic aneurysm screening on mortality in men: a randomised controlled trial. *Lancet* 2002; **360**: 1531–9.
3. Kim LG, Scott RA, Thompson SG, *et al.* Implications of screening for abdominal aortic aneurysms on surgical workload. *Br J Surg* 2005; **92**: 171–6.
4. Wilson WR, Fishwick G, Sir Peter RFB, Thompson MM. Suitability of ruptured AAA for endovascular repair. *J Endovasc Ther* 2004; **11**: 635–40.
5. Boyle JR, Thompson MM. Endovascular abdominal aortic aneurysm repair is less invasive: now we must prove its efficacy. *J Endovasc Ther* 2003; **10**: 16–9.
6. Boyle JR, Goodall S, Thompson JP, Bell PR, Thompson MM. Endovascular AAA repair attenuates the inflammatory and renal responses associated with conventional surgery. *J Endovasc Ther* 2000; **7**: 359–71.
7. Boyle JR, Thompson JP, Thompson MM, *et al.* Improved respiratory function and analgesia control after endovascular AAA repair. *J Endovasc Surg* 1997; **4**: 62–5.
8. Bayly PJ, Matthews JN, Dobson PM, Price ML, Thomas DG. In-hospital mortality from abdominal aortic surgery in Great Britain and Ireland: Vascular Anaesthesia Society audit. *Br J Surg* 2001; **88**: 687–92.
9. Biancari F, Hobo R, Juvonen T. Glasgow Aneurysm Score predicts survival after endovascular stenting of abdominal aortic aneurysm in patients from the EUROSTAR registry. *Br J Surg* 2006; **93**: 191–4.
10. Buth J, van Marrewijk CJ, Harris PL, *et al.* Outcome of endovascular abdominal aortic aneurysm repair in patients with conditions considered unfit for an open procedure: a report on the EUROSTAR experience. *J Vasc Surg* 2002; **35**: 211–21.
11. Harris PL, Vallabhaneni SR, Desgranges P, *et al.* Incidence and risk factors of late rupture, conversion, and death after endovascular repair of infrarenal aortic aneurysms: the EUROSTAR experience. European collaborators on stent/graft techniques for aortic aneurysm repair. *J Vasc Surg* 2000; **32**: 739–49.
12. EVAR trial participants. Endovascular aneurysm repair and outcome in patients unfit for open repair of abdominal aortic aneurysm (EVAR trial 2): randomised controlled trial. *Lancet* 2005; **365**: 2187–92.
13. EVAR trial participants. Endovascular aneurysm repair versus open repair in patients with abdominal aortic aneurysm (EVAR trial 1): randomised controlled trial. *Lancet* 2005; **365**: 2179–86.
14. Greenhalgh RM, Brown LC, Kwong GP, Powell JT, Thompson SG. Comparison of endovascular aneurysm repair with open repair in patients with abdominal aortic aneurysm (EVAR trial 1), 30-day operative mortality results: randomised controlled trial. *Lancet* 2004; **364**: 843–8.

15. Blankensteijn JD, de Jong SE, Prinssen M, *et al*. Two-year outcomes after conventional or endovascular repair of abdominal aortic aneurysms. *N Engl J Med* 2005; **352**: 2398–405.
16. Prinssen M, Verhoeven EL, Buth J, *et al*. A randomized trial comparing conventional and endovascular repair of abdominal aortic aneurysms. *N Engl J Med* 2004; **351**: 1607–18.
17. Lippmann M, Lingam K, Rubin S, Julka I, White R. Anesthesia for endovascular repair of abdominal and thoracic aortic aneurysms: a review article. *J Cardiovasc Surg (Torino)* 2003; **44**: 443–51.
18. Parra JR, Crabtree T, McLafferty RB, *et al*. Anesthesia technique and outcomes of endovascular aneurysm repair. *Ann Vasc Surg* 2005; **19**: 123–9.
19. Verhoeven EL, Cina CS, Tielliu IF, *et al*. Local anesthesia for endovascular abdominal aortic aneurysm repair. *J Vasc Surg* 2005; **42**: 402–9.
20. Veith FJ, Ohki T, Lipsitz EC, Suggs WD, Cynamon J. Treatment of ruptured abdominal aneurysms with stent grafts: a new gold standard? *Semin Vasc Surg* 2003; **16**: 171–5.
21. Huynh TT, Miller CC, III, Estrera AL, *et al*. Correlations of cerebrospinal fluid pressure with hemodynamic parameters during thoracoabdominal aortic aneurysm repair. *Ann Vasc Surg* 2005; **19**: 619–24.
22. Safi HJ, Miller CC III, Huynh TT, *et al*. Distal aortic perfusion and cerebrospinal fluid drainage for thoracoabdominal and descending thoracic aortic repair: ten years of organ protection. *Ann Surg* 2003; **238**: 372–80.
23. Rigberg DA, McGory ML, Zingmond DS, *et al*. Thirty-day mortality statistics underestimate the risk of repair of thoracoabdominal aortic aneurysms: a statewide experience. *J Vasc Surg* 2006; **43**: 217–22.
24. Leurs LJ, Bell R, Degrieck Y, *et al*. Endovascular treatment of thoracic aortic diseases: combined experience from the EUROSTAR and United Kingdom Thoracic Endograft registries. *J Vasc Surg* 2004; **40**: 670–9.
25. Sayed S, Thompson MM. Endovascular repair of the descending thoracic aorta: evidence for the change in clinical practice. *Vascular* 2005; **13**: 148–57.
26. Cho JS, Haider SE, Makaroun MS. US multicenter trials of endoprostheses for the endovascular treatment of descending thoracic aneurysms. *J Vasc Surg* 2006; **43**(Suppl. A): 12A–19A.
27. Makaroun MS, Dillavou ED, Kee ST, *et al*. Endovascular treatment of thoracic aortic aneurysms: results of the phase II multicenter trial of the GORE TAG thoracic endoprosthesis. *J Vasc Surg* 2005; **41**: 1–9.
28. O'Neill S, Greenberg RK, Haddad F, *et al*. Prospective analysis of fenestrated endovascular grafting: intermediate-term outcomes. *Eur J Vasc Endovasc Surg* 2006; **32**: 115–23.
29. Rothwell PM, Eliasziw M, Gutnikov SA, *et al*. Analysis of pooled data from the randomised controlled trials of endarterectomy for symptomatic carotid stenosis. *Lancet* 2003; **361**: 107–16.
30. Young B, Moore WS, Robertson JT, *et al*. An analysis of perioperative surgical mortality and morbidity in the asymptomatic carotid atherosclerosis study. ACAS Investigators: Asymptomatic Carotid Artherosclerosis Study. *Stroke* 1996; **27**: 2216–24.
31. Halliday A, Mansfield A, Marro J, *et al*. Prevention of disabling and fatal strokes by successful carotid endarterectomy in patients without recent neurological symptoms: randomised controlled trial. *Lancet* 2004; **363**: 1491–502.

32. Rerkasem K, Bond R, Rothwell PM. Local versus general anaesthesia for carotid endarterectomy. *Cochrane Database Syst Rev* 2004: CD000126; http://www.wchrane.org/reviews/en/ab000126.html.

33. Yadav JS, Wholey MH, Kuntz RE, *et al*. Protected carotid-artery stenting versus endarterectomy in high-risk patients. *N Engl J Med* 2004; **351**: 1493–501.

34. Yadav JS, Wholey MH, Kuntz RE, *et al*. Endovascular versus surgical treatment in patients with carotid stenosis in the Carotid and Vertebral Artery Transluminal Angioplasty Study (CAVATAS): a randomised trial. *Lancet* 2001; **357**: 1729–37.

35. Brooks WH, McClure RR, Jones MR, Coleman TL, Breathitt L. Carotid angioplasty and stenting versus carotid endarterectomy for treatment of asymptomatic carotid stenosis: a randomized trial in a community hospital. *Neurosurgery* 2004; **54**: 318–24.

36. Naylor AR, Bolia A, Abbott RJ, *et al*. Randomized study of carotid angioplasty and stenting versus carotid endarterectomy: a stopped trial. *J Vasc Surg* 1998; **28**: 326–34.

37. Alos J, Carreno P, Lopez JA, *et al*. Efficacy and safety of sclerotherapy using polidocanol foam: a controlled clinical trial. *Eur J Vasc Endovasc Surg* 2006; **31**: 101–7.

38. Belcaro G, Cesarone MR, Di RA, *et al*. Foam-sclerotherapy, surgery, sclerotherapy, and combined treatment for varicose veins: a 10-year, prospective, randomized, controlled, trial (VEDICO trial). *Angiology* 2003; **54**: 307–15.

39. Guex JJ, Allaert FA, Gillet JL, Chleir F. Immediate and mid-term complications of sclerotherapy: report of a prospective multicenter registry of 12,173 sclerotherapy sessions. *Dermatol Surg* 2005; **31**: 123–8.

40. Mundy L, Merlin TL, Fitridge RA, Hiller JE. Systematic review of endovenous laser treatment for varicose veins. *Br J Surg* 2005; **92**: 1189–94.

41. Min RJ, Khilnani NM. Endovenous laser treatment of saphenous vein reflux. *Tech Vasc Interv Radiol* 2003; **6**: 125–31.

42. Min RJ, Khilnani N, Zimmet SE. Endovenous laser treatment of saphenous vein reflux: long-term results. *J Vasc Interv Radiol* 2003; **14**: 991–6.

Christopher Dodds

CHAPTER

4

Anaesthesia for the elderly

The care of the elderly patient during anaesthesia is one of the most common tasks we perform. It has the highest rate of serious complications and long-term effects and yet it is also the least researched and taught element of anaesthetic practice. The absolute number of the elderly and their relative proportion in our population are increasing and will do so until the latter part of the century. This has an impact not only on the challenges to our anaesthetic practice, but also, because of the reduction in the proportion of people paying taxes, in the country's ability to pay for healthcare. Increased disability and dependence on other carers greatly add to this burden. The figure of a 25% incidence[1] of cognitive dysfunction following major surgery would cause political intervention in any other group of patients. There have been some advances in our understanding of the elderly, in the availability of newer drugs and techniques for instance, that make a review worthwhile.

The basics of getting old

The research into aging and the cellular process underlying[2] these are advancing rapidly in many areas. Integrating these into the responses we observe is more difficult, largely because getting older is a combination of aging at a cellular, organ and systems level with the residual impact of acute and chronic disease states, and finally the adaptation of life-style the patient uses to cope as long as possible. It is this behavioural adaptation that masks many of the underlying processes of importance to us. Vital systems are the most robust, for obvious reasons, and the control of pH, temperature and most fluid volumes

Recent Advances in Anaesthesia and Intensive Care 24, ed. J. N. Cashman and R. M. Grounds.
Published by Cambridge University Press. © Cambridge University Press 2007.

does not change significantly throughout life. Other systems have more striking changes.

Cellular changes

The genetic control of intracellular processes is of importance to us and one of them is the impact that the binding and elimination of β-amyloid that occurs within neurones has on their function. The breakdown of β-amyloid is regulated by the apolipoprotein epsilon (APO E) family of genes. There are four alleles of this gene and each has a different effect on the binding and subsequent removal of β-amyloid. If this process is impaired it builds up within the cell, finally leading to cell death. This is believed to be an underlying cause of much of the dementia seen in clinical practice.

Stem cells are capable of transforming into individual cell lines and are an essential component of repair and recovery from tissue injury. They are still present in muscles in the elderly but usually have lost the ability to be transformed. This results in a progressive loss of myocytes with fatty invasion and fibrosis. The initiation of the process of transformation is largely governed by 'Notch' receptors on the cellular surface of the stem cells. With aging these fail to respond to their normal ligands. Interesting work on rodents has identified that transfusion of blood from young animals into old ones re-activates these stem cells.[3] The active component of the blood has not yet been identified but it does raise the possibility of being able to actively increase the effectiveness of rehabilitation and convalescence in the elderly.

There are changes in the neuraxial skeleton that have important consequences for anaesthesia. These relate to the astrocytic syncitium that envelopes the axons throughout the central nervous system. It is derived from ectodermal cells (as is the retina) and is a potent repair system[4] following neuronal damage. Because the cells are linked as a syncitium, they can transmit chemically mediated messages rapidly throughout the central nervous system (CNS). They have intimate connections with axons through microglia that 'sample' their immediate environment. Following injury they swell, and trigger off several defensive processes[5] such as the induction of nitric oxide synthetase (NOS) and the production of heat-shock proteins.[6] These processes remain active for many months after the injury, if not years. Subsequent oxidative stress (for instance, from a hypoxic episode) will re-start this process, possibly leading to cell apoptosis. There is also a synergy between these dormant mechanisms and the APO gene system. Reactivation triggers β-amyloid production that further increases the risk of cell death.[7]

The astrocyte-based response to an injury such as sectioning of an axon is also age dependent to a degree. Injury to axons within the spinal cord progresses onto attempts to re-establish neuronal conduction between the damaged ends of the neurone. This process in the elderly is restricted because of fibrosis occurring between the damaged ends, effectively leaving a permanent scar. Mediators that may improve this process around the immediate period of injury actually appear harmful only a few days into the injury response process. These insights into the variable response to injury that differ with aging may allow tailored therapy to restore these failing processes of the elderly to that seen in younger patients.

Organ-level changes with aging

These are common across all systems, but for anaesthetists it is the changes in the cardiovascular, respiratory and central nervous systems that have most impact. Some aspects of this have not changed but are often poorly remembered.

Cardiovascular reserve is markedly affected by aging especially if accompanied by a life-style that does not include regular exercise. The progressive myocardial interstitial fibrosis leads to a fall in contractility and increased stiffness of the ventricular walls. This change in compliance affects systolic contraction and diastolic relaxation. It is this delayed diastolic relaxation that reduces the atrial assisted ventricular filling to about 50% of the value in early adulthood, by the age of 80. The cardiac valves become thickened and thrombi develop. This, especially on the left side of the heart, leads to the functional murmurs that are heard in 55% of men aged more than 75 years. Only about 7% of these are owing to a clinically important lesion. Adrenergic sensitivity also changes markedly with a reduced responsiveness of the β-adrenergic receptors to circulating catecholamines. The precise cause of this (decreased affinity, down-regulation or changes in receptor density or transduction) is still unclear.

The respiratory system changes are largely related to a change in the distribution of elastic tissue from the parenchyma of the lungs to the pleura and chest wall. This leads to increasing ability of the small airways to collapse as the residual volume decreases. The increase in this closing volume encroaches on tidal ventilation when supine in most patients over 65 years of age. Any additional respiratory problems (e.g. diffusion problems caused by pulmonary oedema, further shunting from pneumonia or poor cardiac output reducing the mixed venous saturation) can lead to dramatic deterioration in oxygenation.

Systems effects

The most effective systemic process is that of behavioural adaptation to increasingly limited levels of physical activity. This is an invisible process as the patient stops high energy-dependent activities, heavy shopping for instance, and uses carers or relatives to buy for them when doing their own shopping. Failing to enquire about the current activities of daily living will often miss these important clues to actual physical reserve. The limitation of fluid intake because of immobility and a fear of incontinence is another frequent observation.

Pre-anaesthetic considerations

Exercise testing

The changes described above may lead to a failure in the integrated responses to routine tasks, such as exercise, even if this is limited by other disease states such as arthritis. The use of metabolic equivalents (METs) is a common method of estimating oxygen-dependent exercise tolerance. A value of less than 4 is indicative of a rapidly increasing risk of major post-operative complications. Unfortunately, the very group we most need information on is the group that cannot perform these activities, for instance because of joint disease. Drug-induced exercise testing can bridge this gap, but is rarely available on demand.

There is intense interest in cardiopulmonary exercise testing and anaerobic thresholds in the elderly high-risk surgical patient and this can be used even in patients with severe arthritis.[8] The acute optimisation of these patients does improve outcome but this has often been used in the acute setting with little information available to inform us as to whether a more long-term strategy would also provide benefits. There are good examples of the benefits of identifying exercise limitation at an early stage of operative planning, especially for entirely elective surgery, when prescribing an exercise programme can improve overall performance even in the old and unfit.[9]

Medication

Another major problem in the pre-operative assessment of these patients is that of their regular medication. These must include nicotine and alcohol although it is more usual to refer to the prescribed medication for significant medical disorders. The commonest groups are the cardiovascular, psychotropic and endocrine drugs. Compliance is related to both the number of drugs being taken and the frequency of administration. Where more than two drugs are being taken, compliance falls rapidly. The elderly also stop drugs if they (often mistakenly) believe that their deterioration in health may be because of them. A simple list of the drugs prescribed does not at all mean they are actually being taken.

Some of these prescribed drugs are best stopped before surgery but a sizeable number are important to continue. Others require alteration to a parenteral formulation or even a change in drug prior to surgery. The normal time allowed for effective loss of effect is 3–5 times the elimination half-life of the drug (a figure that is very unpredictable in the elderly patient).

Cardiovascular drugs are usually best continued. Cessation causes a time-related increase in complications (> 24 hours equating to a 14% increase and > 48 hours to a 27% increase in non-surgical complications).[10] Some drugs do have rebound effects on withdrawal and these are better continued. The β-blockers are best continued and there is evidence that it may be of benefit to administer them to high-risk cardiovascular patients peri-operatively. Calcium channel-blocking agents have a similar safety profile, with the possible exception of the short-acting (and sympathetic stimulating) agents such as nifedepine. Exceptions are the ACE inhibitors and angiotensin II receptor antagonists (such as losartan or candesartan). Both groups of drugs have a risk of unpredictable, severe and occasionally refractive hypotension on induction of anaesthesia. They are better avoided on the day of surgery.

Psychotropic drugs are very commonly used in the elderly, and include the benzodiazepines and the tricyclic antidepressants used for chronic pain states. There do not appear to be major problems with these drugs but they are often stopped prior to surgery. The monoamine oxidase inhibitors are traditionally stopped and opiates such as pethidine avoided. The newer, more specific agents are often given in sufficiently high doses to lose this specificity and should be regarded as much the same risk as the older drugs.

Anti-Parkinsonian medication should not be stopped, and may need to be given during the procedure if the devastating rigidity or risk of the neuro-leptic syndrome is to be avoided. The patients are often very expert at the timing and combinations of drugs to suit their condition and this should be identified and adhered to.

Frailty

This embodies the concept that some older patients become increasingly vulnerable to, for instance, surgical stress, because they have run out of physiological reserve in many organ systems[11] and are generally incapable of maintaining the high level of metabolic demand that surgery triggers in patients.[12] These patients are at a very high risk for developing postoperative complications including death. They can be recognised by their appearance (thin, pale, often with a 'vague' affect and accompanied by carers or other relatives). This group of patients should be offered the most minimally invasive procedures balanced against the likelihood of long-term benefit of more major surgery.

Per-operative considerations

Drug-handling changes

The majority of changes seen in the elderly are owing to alterations in pharmaco-kinetics rather than dynamics. There is a loss of muscle cell mass and a proportionate increase in body fat. These cause a fall in total body water. An alteration in the distribution of lipophilic and hydrophilic drugs is predictable but more difficult to quantitate. Cardiac output falls and the muscles are no longer vessel rich. This accounts for the slow onset, prolonged action and incomplete reversal of the neuromuscular blocking agents. This is less pronounced with the benzylisoquinolones, such as atracurium, than the aminosteroids.[13]

Volatile agents

The MAC (minimum alveolar concentration) falls with age and that for Desflurane halves with aging from 10% in young children to 5% in the over 65-year-olds. The benefit of the poorly lipid soluble agents (Sevoflurane and Desflurane) is in their rapid and almost complete recovery profile.[14] The residual attenuation of hypoxic and hypercarbic drives seen with the more soluble older agents is largely avoided. Problems with coughing and airway irritation are less in the elderly and this make the choice of agent more straightforward.

Hypnotic agents

Benzodiazepines have a prolonged action in the elderly. Midazolam has about a four-fold reduction in dosing requirement by the age of 80. Its clearance falls to 30% of the value aged 20 and its context-sensitive half-times double by the age of 80. Diazepam's metabolites include desmethyldiazepam, which has more depressant activity than the parent drug. It also has a very long half-life of up to 190 hours.

Propofol is approximately 30% more potent by the age of 90. There are also changes in clearance, rapidly equilibrating volume and clearance between compartments. One effect is to prolong recovery from long (over four hours) infusions by 100%.

Opioids

Remifentanil has a clear place in the elderly despite it being twice as potent in the elderly, yet largely retains its rate of clearance by plasma esterases. This makes recovery as fast as in young patients although there is a larger variability.

Monitoring

Trans-oesophageal echocardiography has proved an invaluable monitor in high risk cardiac and vascular surgery. Data on outcomes in the elderly are rare at present.

Postoperative care

Acute pain management

Acute pain management in the elderly is still poor, prompting the UK Department of Health's National Service Framework for Older People[15] to identify effective pain control in several of its 'standards'. Cognitively intact patients can report and score their pain effectively with either verbal or numeric scales. Visual scales are confusing and unreliable.[16] Those with a cognitive dysfunction still perceive pain but may not be able to remember the avoidance strategies to reduce the pain, of a fracture for instance. Behavioural markers often do allow a judgement to be made even in severely demented patients.

Communication difficulties, owing to either vocabulary changes or failure of special senses, vision or hearing, all make assessment more difficult especially in a noisy ward. While younger patients are often thought to over-estimate their pain, they do get prescribed effective doses of analgesics, whilst the elderly are believed to often understate their pain but are still prescribed ineffective doses of analgesia, usually for fear of respiratory depression. Trauma patients often only receive simple analgesics rather than opioids, despite these published standards.

Cognitive dysfunction after surgery

The incidence of this remains very high and it may present either acutely as delirium or become apparent several days after surgery as postoperative cognitive dysfunction.

Delirium

Delirium is occasionally unavoidable but it is one of the causes of postoperative confusional states. The others include psychosis, dementia and drug withdrawal. It is a transient mental condition[17,18] that has a global disorder of cognition (thinking, perception, memory) and attention (alertness, selectiveness or directiveness). It is a common condition, especially in older patients during an acute illness. After the age of 70, it may affect up to 24% of emergency medical admissions[19] and is even more common after surgery[20] when it may affect over 35% of patients. It has a marked impact on morbidity and mortality in these patients. It characteristically has a sudden onset, a variable or fluctuating severity and a marked effect on the sleep/wake cycle. Patients may be agitated or more rarely 'quiet'. This latter group are often missed. There is a definition of delirium based on the Diagnostic and Statistical Manual of Mental Disorders (DSM IV)[21] which identifies three patterns: substance intoxications, multiple aetiologies and general medical conditions. It is the latter that is the most common post-operatively. Previously identified cognitive impairment, extreme old age, severity of illness and psychoactive drug usage are important predisposing factors.

Delirium is believed to be an acute cholinergic disorder and may be precipitated by many drugs but especially the centrally acting anticholinergic drugs such as atropine. Metabolic stress, hypoxia or hypoglycaemia, are other potent precipitating factors. Avoidance of known triggers/risks has been tried in patients who are at risk, but to date has been disappointingly ineffective. Treatment depends on eliminating known triggers, such as infection, metabolic factors etc., and then instituting drug therapy. Good nursing care and a well-lit environment may reduce the episodes of agitation, and limiting the number of carers or using relatives may also be effective. If not then drug therapy will be necessary. Benzodiazepines are more likely to cause respiratory depression, and have very long elimination times. They may also provoke paradoxical agitation in some patients. Haloperidol is the most commonly prescribed drug and should be given in a high enough dosage to be effective, but no more. It should be given for a few days (until control is assured) and then slowly withdrawn. It does have a wide variety of side-effects and these should be monitored, especially QTc prolongation (QTc is the rate-related interval and is a more sensitive marker of the risk of arrhythmia than simple measurement of the QT interval).

There are other drugs that are effective but these should usually be given under the guidance of a psychiatrist.

Postoperative cognitive dysfunction

Postoperative cognitive dysfunction (POCD) is one of the most common complications of major surgery in the over-65 population, with an incidence of about 25%. This figure has not changed for over 50 years[22] despite all the advances in monitoring, in agents and in surgical and anaesthetic techniques.

Postoperative cognitive dysfunction is characterised by memory impairment, failure of executive functioning (planning/organization etc.), and attention or speed of information processing and language impairment. More subtle changes in social dysinhibition are also common. It is more likely in patients with a previous episode of delirium, known cognitive impairment, age over 75, those having a second procedure, or who have had prolonged anaesthesia. Some procedures are particularly high risk, such as cardiac procedures under bypass, neurosurgical and major abdominal procedures. Despite many very large studies to try to identify, for instance, if regional techniques are more protective than general anaesthesia or whether hypoxia or hypotension were causative, no clear answer has been found.

Although POCD is believed to be a cholinergic failure within the CNS, the use of cognitive-enhancing drugs (such as those used for dementia) has not been to any advantage. One possible avenue for research is investigations into the interaction between the astrocyte activation following neuronal injury that lasts for several months if not years, and the predisposition that this astrocyte activation has for damage by a subsequent oxidative stress. Many volatile and intravenous anaesthetic agents have actions on neuronal[23,24,25] receptors, ranging from NMDA (N-methyl-D-aspartate) to cholinergic and adrenergic receptors. Some of these actions are protective and others, depending on the concentration and the presence of mild hypoxia, are damaging. At present it is difficult to identify in vitro whether such damage has occurred but this may provide a plausible reason for the apparent lack of association between hypoxia or hypotension and subsequent POCD. Work on pre-conditioning neuronal receptors with volatile anaesthetics is underway and producing some promising results that may lead to strategies for those patients who have already been identified as high risk.

Summary

There are significant advances in related research fields to anaesthesia that may provide insights into the remaining major problems with caring for elderly patients. Some are owing to better drugs, to better equipment and monitoring, whilst others are owing to developments in the underlying cell biology. We are beginning to understand the underlying processes that may lead to cognitive dysfunction and, with that, the hope of avoidance or even pre-emptive medication to preserve mental function. It may be that within five years we will be able to review the provision of anaesthesia for the elderly and dismiss as historical some of the most important aspects of care today.

References

1. Rasmussen LS, Johnson T, Kuipers HM, *et al*. ISPOCD2 (International Study of Postoperative Cognitive Dysfunction) Investigators. Does anaesthesia cause postoperative cognitive dysfunction? A randomised study of regional versus general anaesthesia in 438 elderly patients. *Acta Anaesthesiol Scand* 2003; **47**: 260–6.
2. Wright WE, Shay JW. Telomere biology in aging and cancer. *J Am Geriatr Soc* 2005; **53**(9 Suppl.): S292–S4.
3. Conboy IM, Conboy MJ, Wagers AJ, *et al*. Rejuvenation of aged progenitor cells by exposure to a young systemic environment. *Nature* 2005; **433**: 760–4.
4. Aldskogius H, Kozlova EN. Central neuron–glial and glial–glial interactions following axon injury. *Progress Neurobiol* 1998; **55**: 1–26.
5. Griffin, WS. Inflammation and neurodegenerative diseases. *Am J Clin Nutr* 2006; **83**: 470S–4S.
6. Acarin L, Paris J, Gonzalez B, Castellano B. Glial expression of small heat shock proteins following an excitotoxic lesion in the immature rat brain. *Glia* 2002; **38**: 1–14.
7. Abildstrom H, Christiansen M, Siersma VD, Rasmussen LS. Apolipoprotein E genotype and cognitive dysfunction after noncardiac surgery. *Anesthesiology* 2004; **101**: 855–61.
8. Philbin, EF, Ries, MD, French, TS. Feasibility of maximal cardiopulmonary exercise testing in patients with end-stage arthritis of the hip and knee prior to total joint arthroplasty. *Chest* 1995; **108**: 174–81.
9. Kennedy JM, van Rij AM, Spears GF *et al*. Polypharmacy in a general surgical unit and consequences of drug withdrawal. *Br J Clin Pharm* 2000; **49**: 353–62.
10. Ades, PA, Waldmann, ML, Poehlman, ET *et al*. Exercise conditioning in older coronary patients. Submaximal lactate response and endurance capacity. *Circulation* 1993; **88**: 572–7.
11. Ehsani AA, Spina RJ, Peterson LR *et al*. Attenuation of cardiovascular adaptations to exercise in frail octogenarians. *J Appl Physiol* 2003; **95**: 1781–8.
12. Rockwood K, Mtinski AB, MacKnight C. Some mathematical models of frailty and their clinical implications. *Age Ageing* 2004; **33**: 430–2.
13. Cope TM, Hunter JM. Selecting neuromuscular-blocking drugs for elderly patients. *Drugs Ageing* 2003; **20**: 125–40.
14. Bennett JA, Lingaraju N, Horrow JC, McElrath T, Keykhah MM. Elderly patients recover more rapidly from desflurane than from isoflurane anesthesia. *J Clin Anesth* 1992; **4**: 378–81.
15. *NSF for Older People: Medicines and Older People Appendix*. London: DoH; 2001; available at: http://www.dh.gov.uk/assetRoot/04/06/72/47/04067247.pdf.

16. Briggs M, Closs JS. A descriptive study of the use of visual analogue scales and verbal rating scales for the assessment of postoperative pain in orthopedic patients. *J Pain Symptom Managem* 1999; **18**: 438–46.

17. Lipowski ZJ. Delirium (acute confusional states). *JAMA* 1987; **258**: 1789–92.

18. Lipowski ZJ. Delirium in the elderly patient. *N Engl J Med* 1989; **320**: 578–82.

19. Naughton BJ, Moran MB, Kadah H, Heman-Ackah Y, Longano J. Delirium and other cognitive impairments in older adults in an emergency department. *Ann Emerg Med* 1995; **25**: 751–5.

20. Inouye SK. Delirium in hospitalized older patients. *Clin Geriatr Med* 1998; **14**: 745–64.

21. American Psychiatric Association. *Diagnostic and Statistical Manual of Mental Disorders*, 4th edn. Washington DC: American Psychiatric Association, 1994.

22. Bedford PD. Adverse cerebral effects of anaesthesia on old people. *Lancet* 1955; **269**: 259–63.

23. Jevtovic-Todorovic V, Carter LB. The anesthetics nitrous oxide and ketamine are more neurotoxic to old than to young rat brain. *Neurobiol Aging* 2005; **26**: 947–56.

24. Butterfield NN, Graf P, Ries CR, MacLeod BA. The effect of repeated isoflurane anesthesia on spatial and psychomotor performance in young and aged mice. *Anesth Analg* 2004; **98**: 1305–11.

25. Shinozaki M, Usui Y, Yamaguchi S, Okuda Y, Kitajima T. Recovery of psychomotor function after propofol sedation is prolonged in the elderly. *Can J Anaesth* 2002; **49**: 927–31.

Anthony Gray

Deaths following anaesthesia: lessons from NCEPOD

Death is the ultimate unfavourable outcome after anaesthesia. The first anaesthetic death has been reported as that of Alexis Montigny in Auxerre on 10th July 1847 from respiratory obstruction owing to the administration of ether.[1] Deaths such as this that are directly caused by the anaesthetic process ('direct anaesthetic deaths') are obviously of great concern but deaths where anaesthetic factors contribute to a patient's death in combination with factors related to the patient's condition and to the surgery ('anaesthetic-related deaths') are equally important. Anaesthetic-related deaths are more common, so improvements in this area will have the greater impact on the overall burden of morbidity and mortality.

Anaesthetic mortality rate

Studies of the rates of death following anaesthesia have two uses. Patients perceive anaesthesia to be inherently dangerous and want to know the risks of dying under anaesthesia: conversely anaesthetists want to know about mortality rates to defend themselves against unwarranted attacks on the safety of their specialty. Secondly anaesthetists need repeated studies on anaesthetic mortality to measure whether efforts to improve anaesthetic safety have borne fruit. There have been many studies of anaesthetic mortality over the last 50 years. Unfortunately comparisons between studies are problematic. The definition of an anaesthetic death, the time period within which the patient died, the classification of the extent of anaesthetic involvement in the patient's death and the type of study population all vary from one study to another. Because of these differences it is difficult to be certain that mortality rates are improving; nor is it easy to know how the

Recent Advances in Anaesthesia and Intensive Care 24, ed. J. N. Cashman and R. M. Grounds.
Published by Cambridge University Press. © Cambridge University Press 2007.

results of published studies should be extrapolated to the circumstances of an individual patient seeking advice about anaesthetic risks.

The patient information leaflet[2] published under the auspices of the Royal College of Anaesthetists quotes the Confidential Enquiry into Perioperative Deaths (CEPOD) report published in 1987[3] for deaths directly related to anaesthesia. The study population consisted of all patients operated on in three of the 13 regional health authorities in England at that time and derived a figure of 1:185 000. There is a belief that anaesthesia has become safer still since the 1970s and anaesthesia is held up as a model for improving patient safety that other specialties should emulate.[4] Medical indemnity organisations class anaesthetists as at medium risk for claims rather than among those at the highest risk, as in the past.

The experience of Gibbs and the Western Australian Anaesthetic Mortality Committee is helpful.[5] This study is unusual because it is a continuous longitudinal study that has collected data since 1980, and the definitions and classifications have remained largely unchanged throughout. Deaths directly related to anaesthesia ('anaesthesia as the primary cause') correspond to Category I as defined by Edwards in 1956:[6] 'Where it was reasonably certain that death was caused by the anaesthetic agent or technique of administration, or in other ways coming entirely within the anaesthetist's province'. 'Anaesthesia-related' deaths also include Edward's Categories II and III: that is, deaths where anaesthesia was a contributing cause but there was some element of doubt as to whether the anaesthetic was entirely responsible; and cases where both anaesthetic and surgical factors were involved. The results show that the anaesthetic mortality rate fell during the early part of the 1980s and has remained relatively stable since (Table 5.1).

Table 5.1 Anaesthesia mortality rates in Western Australia, 1980–2002.

Report period (years)	Number of deaths with anaesthesia as the primary cause	Total number of anaesthesia-related deaths	Annual rate of anaesthesia-related deaths per million population	Annual rate of anaesthesia-related deaths per 100 000 surgical procedures
1980–1984	24	39	5.8	6.5
1985–1987	4	5	1.1	1.2
1988–1990	6	9	1.9	1.7
1991–1993	14	16	3.2	2.5
1994–1996	14	19	3.6	2.9
1997–1999	6	11	2.0	1.3
2000–2002	2	16	2.9	1.7

The study population was 1.93 million in 2002 and the number of surgical procedures was 321 400 but the number of anaesthesia-related deaths over the years have been small, so any conclusions about trends in mortality must be guarded. It would appear that direct anaesthetic deaths are now very rare (but do still happen). Most deaths occur in circumstances where anaesthesia is one of a number of factors contributing to the patient's death.

As well as mortality rates, studies have looked at the causes of anaesthesia-related deaths. The findings are not surprising. Causes have been quoted as inadequate preparation and failures in monitoring,[7] respiratory and medication-related events,[8] and cardiovascular management.[8] A persistent finding is that anaesthesia-related deaths are more common in patients who have a higher American Society of Anesthesiologists (ASA) score.[7,8,9] This may be because the management of such patients is more complex so that errors are more likely, or it may be that sicker patients are less able to tolerate the consequences of such errors. These data qualify the findings of Eichhorn[10] in 1989. The statistic that 319 000 anaesthetics were administered between 1985 and 1988 at the component hospitals of the Harvard Department of Anaesthesia without a major preventable intra-operative anaesthetic injury is often quoted as evidence of the safety of current anaesthesia. However, patients had to have an ASA score of only 1 or 2 to be included in the study population. This paper does not provide evidence for the safety of anaesthesia for patients of ASA 3, 4 or 5, in whom adverse outcomes are more likely.

Not everyone is convinced that anaesthetic mortality is improving. Lagasse[11] carried out a combination of literature review and examination of original data from two hospital networks in the USA. He concluded that during the 1990s anaesthetic-related mortality was stable at a rate of 7.7 per 100 000 anaesthetics, considerably higher than the rate reported by Gibbs. In support, the report by Braz[7] in 2006 from a tertiary teaching centre in Brazil found an anaesthesia-related mortality rate of 11.2 per 100 000 anaesthetics. Cooper and Gaba[12], in an editorial on the paper by Lagasse, argued that the gains in the safety of anaesthesia over five decades were real but stressed that the struggle for safety is never-ending. It is possible that efforts have reached a plateau in the last 15 years. Therefore, what other sources can anaesthetists use to help improve patient outcome?

Factors influencing patient outcome

The NCEPOD (National Confidential Enquiry into Patient Outcome and Death), the successor to CEPOD, has never repeated the calculation of a mortality rate as performed by CEPOD; it was recognised that there were problems in assuring the accuracy of both numerator and denominator figures. Instead NCEPOD adopted a protocol to examine the quality of the delivery of care and not specifically study the causation of death. The fact that NCEPOD was set up as a joint study between anaesthesia and surgery means that it has produced unique insights into the way that poor care can compromise the care of patients.

The first lesson to be learned from NCEPOD's experience is that individuals and departments have to show humility and be open to the possibility that there is room for improvement. Some anaesthetists have been very critical of their own practice. Others have returned questionnaires with comments such as *'This utterly futile audit has taken 1–2 hours of my valuable time. I completely resent this.'* The 2002 NCEPOD report[13] noted that 6% of anaesthetic departments did not have morbidity/mortality review meetings at all, and 57% of all deaths reported did not undergo anaesthetic review. Remediable deficiencies in care will not be found if anaesthetists do not go looking for them. The death of an ASA 2 patient after elective surgery is likely to be unexpected and subject to review; in contrast there may be a temptation to assume that every death in an elderly patient undergoing surgery for fractured neck of femur is inevitable and so no review occurs. The NCEPOD has found that there are many cases where the patient's condition before surgery was indeed poor, but the chances of survival were compromised by poor care by the anaesthetic or surgical team.

The anaesthetist

Cases reported to NCEPOD have consistently caused concern because of the level of training or experience of staff anaesthetising sick patients. In the past trainees have anaesthetised very sick patients, or patients for major surgery, when their time in the specialty suggested that they were too inexperienced for the degree of difficulty of the case. This has been less common in recent years because the workload of cases not anaesthetised by consultants has shifted from trainees to staff grade and associate specialist (SAS) doctors. The lack of uniformity in the experience and training of doctors entering these posts makes it difficult to judge in a particular case whether an SAS doctor was the right person to be looking after that patient. The NCEPOD found that many SAS doctors who had anaesthetised patients who had subsequently died within 30 days, did not have postgraduate qualifications in anaesthesia. It is debatable how far extra experience in the specialty can compensate for the lack of a postgraduate qualification. This is not to denigrate SAS doctors; it is a plea for anaesthetic departments to ensure that SAS doctors, like trainees, are allocated cases that they are judged competent to manage and feel confident in so doing.

What about the competence of consultants? In the past it has been assumed that as a result of their completion of training and their extended experience, a consultant would be able to manage any case successfully. This is now under question. Many consultants do not receive regular exposure to all types of patients. Data from the report *Extremes of Age*[14] showed that even in 1998 58% of consultant anaesthetists never anaesthetised a child under the age of 6 months. The figure is probably higher now. This may mean such consultants feel themselves lacking the necessary skills if they are called to resuscitate an infant in an emergency. The 2002 NCEPOD report found that a significant number of intensive therapy units (ITUs) had less than ten funded consultant ITU sessions per week. This supports anecdotal evidence that there are still hospitals where Critical Care is covered by anaesthetists who do not have a regular commitment to the specialty. The report on abdominal aortic aneurysm (AAA) surgery[15] found that 22% of elective AAA patients were cared for by anaesthetists who performed less than five AAA elective cases a year. For AAA cases admitted as an emergency 61% of patients were cared for by an anaesthetist who performed less than five emergency AAA cases a year. One-third of the emergency admission patients had an unruptured aneurysm so there might have been an opportunity for the operation to be scheduled when an experienced vascular anaesthetist could be present (see also Chapter 3). These findings show that the trend throughout medicine towards sub-specialisation is being reflected in anaesthesia. Consultants are now responsible, especially out of hours, for cases that they rarely see in their regular work.

Anaesthetists must recognise the wider context of these concerns. Evidence was presented in the AAA report, that for many major operations the greater the volume of cases done by a hospital the lower the patient mortality.[16] This effect could be distinguished from the similar phenomenon, that the greater the volume of cases done by a surgeon the lower the patient mortality.[17] The relative contribution of hospital volume and surgeon volume on overall mortality varied between different operations. The beneficial effects of greater hospital volume will of course include the impact of anaesthetists being more familiar with the anaesthetic implications of the surgery being undertaken. Other elements such as the impact of critical care services will also be significant. Kahn and colleagues[18] found that mechanical ventilation of patients in a hospital with a high case volume was associated with reduced mortality. Given the published evidence, anaesthetic departments have a responsibility to organise their working practices so that wherever possible patients are cared for by anaesthetists who have frequent exposure to the major surgery being undertaken, in hospitals that perform an adequate number of cases. In some cases this may mean accepting that surgery should be moved to another hospital in order to improve patient outcome.

The anaesthetic

Surprisingly, NCEPOD did not find a large number of cases where the intra-operative anaesthetic management of the patient was judged to have compromised the patient's outcome. (The NCEPOD is aware that not all relevant perioperative deaths have been reported to them. Anaesthetists may have been inhibited from reporting deaths when there were major anaesthetic problems.) The chief concern identified by NCEPOD regarding the management of the anaesthetic itself has been the management of regional anaesthesia, especially in combination with general anaesthesia. Clinicians believe that regional anaesthesia, especially the use of postoperative epidural analgesia after elective major surgery, has a beneficial effect on outcome, although the evidence base is not extensive. Similarly, evidence from clinical trials to support the concerns of NCEPOD advisors about the conduct of regional anaesthesia is lacking. However it has been difficult for NCEPOD to ignore cases where this technique was used intra-operatively, in septic and poorly resuscitated emergency patients, who subsequently had systolic blood pressures of 50–70 mmHg for an extended period of time. Such cases should be managed by experienced staff with consideration given to the use of monitoring of central venous pressure and cardiac output.

Preoperative management

Of course anaesthetists do not work on their own, but interact with other specialties and with other clinical professionals. The process starts with preoperative preparation. To compensate for the reduced time between admission and surgery, patients are being seen in pre-admission assessment clinics some days before admission. Unfortunately there is often limited anaesthetic input into these clinics. From the 2002 report, 356 patients were admitted electively or as day cases. These were all patients who died within three days of surgery but only 66% were seen in a pre-assessment clinic. Of these 356 only 18% appeared to have been seen by an anaesthetist. The majority of patients were seen by a nurse practitioner or a surgical house officer or senior house officer. From the AAA report 21% of the 428 patients admitted electively were not seen in a pre-admission assessment clinic. Of the 339 patients who were seen, for 102 patients the most senior doctor carrying out the assessment was a pre-registration house officer. Anaesthetists should ensure that they contribute fully to the pre-admission process. It frustrates the pre-assessment process if surgery is cancelled when the anaesthetist sees the patient for the first time on admission and then perceives the patient to be unfit for operation. Anaesthetists should help establish protocols so that pre-assessment staff know which patients should be seen by an anaesthetist. Departments should ensure that anaesthetic staff of appropriate seniority attend pre-assessment clinics, and that trainees receive teaching and experience in this area of anaesthetic practice. Anaesthetic review of deaths after anaesthesia should include a judgement on whether the pre-assessment process worked properly or whether it could be improved to the advantage of future patients.

Obviously there is much less time for pre-operative assessment and optimisation when a patient is admitted as an emergency. Nevertheless NCEPOD has seen many cases where despite the urgency of the patient's surgical condition there was time to improve their overall status, but this opportunity was spurned; the patient was submitted to anaesthesia and surgery and their outcome was prejudiced by their state at induction. If the patient is very sick it may be sensible to involve critical care physicians before surgery to assist in the optimisation of the patient's condition, with admission to critical care facilities and supervision of resuscitation by intensivists. However, if the patient remains on the ward for preoperative treatment, is this solely a surgical matter, or does the anaesthetist bear some responsibility for satisfactory preoperative preparation? Is it more important to ensure that the patient receives the best management than to argue about whose job it is to carry out a particular task? Or if the anaesthetist does become involved in some way, is there a risk that nothing will actually be done, because the surgeon and the anaesthetist each think that the other will do what is needed?

Whilst criticising clinicians who take patients to theatre in a precipitate manner, NCEPOD has found that other patients have suffered because of delays in their surgical treatment, as have other investigators. A study by Pearse and colleagues of patients scheduled for emergency surgery[19] found considerable delays in more than half. One cause of delay is the unavailability of emergency CEPOD theatres. One of the earliest NCEPOD recommendations was that emergency operating facilities should be available 24 hours a day, but the AAA report found that in 2004 20% of hospitals did not provide CEPOD lists. It is extraordinary that whilst the majority of trusts have provided the resources for proper emergency operating facilities, others do not believe that the care of emergency patients is a priority. Another cause of delay is the failure of junior medical staff to appreciate the severity of a patient's condition, or to ask for assistance from a senior colleague to assess a patient or to expedite their treatment. The NCEPOD considered delays occurred because hospital staff assumed that once emergency patients had been admitted to hospital the need for urgency had passed although it was clear that this was not so. Anaesthetists were involved in some of the delays. Investigations were ordered at the instigation of the anaesthetist which were not strictly necessary, or there was confusion as to who was to decide that the patient was now fit for surgery so the date for surgery was constantly deferred. If the anaesthetist decides that a delay is necessary, how much responsibility does he bear to expedite the investigation or treatment necessary and to confirm that it is now safe to take the patient to theatre, or can that responsibility be left with the surgical team?

Postoperative management

The data returned to NCEPOD illustrate that there are many problems in the postoperative period as well. In some instances trainees over-estimated their abilities and continued to provide inadequate treatment for patients when they should have realised that they needed senior advice. This failure should in part be laid at the door of the trainees, but their supervising consultants were also at fault. It is the duty of the consultant to ensure junior staff know that they should have no inhibitions about calling for senior help and consultants should make themselves aware of the actions of their juniors. The lack of supervision of two senior house officers (SHOs) employed by Southampton General Hospital when a 31-year-old died after routine surgery led to the successful prosecution of the hospital under the UK Health & Safety Act.[20] The NCEPOD has also seen these failings in medical specialties as reported in 2005 in *An Acute Problem*.[21]

The NCEPOD has identified problems with the postoperative management of fluid therapy in successive reports. Some patients received inadequate amounts of fluid and suffered from hypotension, oliguria and renal failure. Others received excessive amounts of fluid with subsequent respiratory and cardiac problems. It is difficult to achieve the correct balance in an elderly, sick patient with co-morbidities – another reason for trainees to seek senior help. However, there is evidence that fluid management was not given proper priority. It is impossible to prescribe rational fluid therapy without knowing the patient's fluid intake and output, but fluid charts that were meant to be returned to NCEPOD were often missing, poorly completed, or merely noted as 'wet bed'. Doctors should ensure that nursing staff keep good records of fluid intake and output. They should also ensure that incontinent patients are catheterised to permit accurate measurement of urine output and to preserve the patients' dignity.

Do anaesthetists have any responsibility for this? It is customary for the theatre anaesthetist to write up fluids for the patient for their return to the ward. Should the anaesthetist visit the ward at the end of the list, or the next day, to check that the fluid status and urine output are satisfactory? What should they do if they are not? Does the anaesthetist have an added responsibility if he has inserted an epidural catheter, given that this may make fluid management more difficult? The AAA study found that in 16% of elective cases when an epidural catheter had been inserted, the anaesthetist could not say when the catheter was removed. This suggests that the anaesthetist had ceased to make postoperative visits and that no robust mechanism was in place to supervise the conduct of postoperative epidural analgesia. What responsibility does the anaesthetist have for care after surgery? Can the anaesthetist walk away if one of his patients suffers inadequate care later in their hospital stay?

Critical care

The relationship with critical care is vital. From the 2002 report 43% of patients were admitted to an intensive therapy (ITU) or high-dependency (HDU) unit after operation. Admission was clinically indicated in another 6% but did not happen, usually because of a shortage of beds. It is important that there is proper consultant input into the care of patients once in critical care. The 2005 report collected data on medical admissions to intensive care and found that 24% of patients had not been reviewed by a consultant intensivist within 12 hours of admission to the unit; some had still not been reviewed after 24 hours. There is no reason to believe that surgical admissions would receive more prompt attention. Anaesthetists must ensure that their trusts provide the resources so that the sickest patients in the hospital can receive consultant review in a timely manner.

An Acute Problem? also highlighted that 46% of medical referrals to ITU were made by SHOs or specialist registrars in year 1 or 2, and the corresponding figure for the ITU doctor accepting the referral was 15%.[21] Approximately a third of cases were referred without the knowledge of the consultant in charge of the case and a third were accepted without any consultant intensivist involvement. Admission to critical care is a serious treatment decision. The patient will be subjected to active, invasive and possibly undignified treatment; this may not be in their best interests when their previous health and their prospects of returning to a good quality of life are considered. There has been ample evidence to NCEPOD over successive reports of patients' care being affected by the inability to supply a critical care bed when required. Giving an ITU bed to one patient can mean denying that bed to another. Obviously the figures above for medical admissions cannot be transferred directly to the surgical setting but they do indicate that anaesthetists should ensure that decisions to refer and admit to critical care are taken by clinicians of appropriate seniority and experience. The 2001 report[22] pointed out that in many cases it is best to refer the patient to critical care before operation. A decision before surgery that postoperative admission to critical care is not in the patient's interest will be very helpful in deciding how best to plan the overall management of the patient.

Patients undergoing surgery are often referred to the medical team, either for advice on the optimisation of concurrent medical conditions before surgery or for help with postoperative complications. Surgeons and anaesthetists expect that the referral will bring extra knowledge and experience to the management of the patient's medical condition, but this is not always so. Cases have been reported to NCEPOD where sick surgical patients were seen by a medical SHO or an inexperienced medical registrar. In other cases advice was received from an experienced registrar, but over the telephone without the physician seeing the patient in person. The anaesthetist must assess the perioperative experience of the physician when judging their opinion. The experience of NCEPOD is that, on occasions, physicians can misinterpret the clinical situation to the detriment of the patient. The way to maximise the benefit of a medical referral is partly in the hands of the surgical team. It has already been highlighted that many perioperative deaths are not subject to review by anaesthetists. When a review does take place, how often are the physicians who may have been involved in the case invited to participate? Unless physicians join in the audit of perioperative deaths they will be unable to reflect on their input into a case and cannot take measures to correct any deficiencies identified.

The patient

There is one other cause of perioperative death to consider: that the patient's condition was so poor before surgery that there was no prospect of the patient surviving. The NCEPOD has counselled on many occasions against performing futile surgery despite pressure to operate from other health workers or the patient's relatives. It is recognised that these judgements are easier to make in hindsight but the vignettes in the NCEPOD reports show that in too many cases it should have been clear at the outset that operation was not in the patient's best interests. Defining the patient's best interests may of course be problematic. It used to be that anaesthetist and surgeon judged surgery to be a success if the patient was alive at the end of the operation. Now that resuscitation and anaesthesia have advanced, patients who would have died on the table can survive to be admitted to ITU, albeit receiving mechanical ventilation and inotropic support. If patients survive for a few days after surgery but do not live to leave hospital, is that in their best interests? Even if the patient leaves hospital, what will their quality of life be after discharge? Evidence is accumulating that ITU survivors suffer from cognitive and physiological disorders and impaired quality of life.[23,24,25] Doctors have a duty to use health care resources wisely.[26] Operating on patients who have no realistic chance of a good outcome denies resources to other patients who would benefit, especially if postoperative care involves the use of critical care facilities. Even if the outlook is not completely hopeless, considerable resources will have been consumed caring for all the patients who did not survive to achieve one patient discharged from hospital. Should this be a consideration?

Conclusion

On the horizon are developments that may allow anaesthetists to modify the long-term health of their patients by the application of new knowledge about the role of inflammation in acute and chronic illness[27] and the influence of genomics in the perioperative period.[28] In the meantime the reports that have been published by NCEPOD identify where anaesthetists can achieve the best outcome possible for their patients by eliminating deficiencies in their own practice and by working together with their colleagues in other specialties. The evidence shows that deaths solely owing to anaesthesia are now very rare, but have not been eliminated completely. It requires all of us to be obsessional about our practice lest complacency leads to a resurgence of avoidable deaths.

References

1. Adams N. The first anaesthetic deaths. *CPD Anaesthesia* 1999; **1**: 142–6.
2. White S. Risks associated with your anaesthetic. Section 14: Death or brain damage. 2006. Royal College of Anaesthetists. Available from http://www.rcoa.ac.uk/docs/death%20or%20brain%20damage.pdf.
3. Buck N, Devlin HB, Lunn JN (eds). *The Report of the Confidential Enquiry into Perioperative Deaths*. London: The Nuffield Provincial Hospitals Trust/ Kings Fund 1987.
4. Gaba DM. Anaesthesiology as a model for patient safety in health care. *BMJ* 2000; **320**: 785–8.
5. Gibbs N, Rodoreda P. Anaesthetic mortality rates in Western Australia. *Anaesth Intensive Care* 2005; **33**: 616–22.
6. Edwards G, Morton HJV, Pask EA, Wylie WD. Deaths associated with anaesthesia. A report on 1,000 cases. *Anaesthesia* 1956; **11**: 194–220.
7. Braz LG, Módolo NSP, do Nascimento P Jr, *et al*. Perioperative cardiac arrest: a study of 53 718 anaesthetics over 9 years from a Brazilian teaching hospital. *Br J Anaesth* 2006; **96**: 569–75.
8. Arbous MS, Grobbee DE, van Kleef JW, *et al*. Mortality associated with anaesthesia: a qualitative analysis to identify risk factors. *Anaesthesia* 2001; **56**: 1141–53.

9. Biboulet P, Aubas P, Dubourdieu J, *et al*. Fatal and non-fatal cardiac arrests related to anesthesia. *Can J Anesth* 2001; **48**: 326–32.

10. Eichhorn JH. Prevention of intra-operative anesthesia accidents and related severe injury through safety monitoring. *Anesthesiology* 1989; **70**: 572–7.

11. Lagasse RS. Anesthesia safety: model or myth? *Anesthesiology* 2002; **97**: 1609–17.

12. Cooper JB, Gaba D. No myth: anesthesia is a model for addressing patient safety (editorial). *Anesthesiology* 2002; **97**: 1335–7.

13. NCEPOD. *Functioning as a Team?* The 2002 report of the National Confidential Enquiry into Perioperative Deaths. London: NCEPOD, 2002. www.ncepod.org.uk

14. NCEPOD. *Extremes of Age*. The 1999 report of the National Confidential Enquiry into Perioperative Deaths. London: NCEPOD, 1999. www.ncepod.org.uk

15. NCEPOD. *Abdominal Aortic Aneurysm: A Service in Need of Surgery?* London: NCEPOD, 2005. www.ncepod.org.uk

16. Birkmeyer JD, Siewers AE, Finlayson EVA, *et al*. Hospital volume and surgical mortality in the United States. *N Engl J Med* 2002; **346**: 1128–37.

17. Birkmeyer JD, Stukel TA, Siewers AE, *et al*. Surgeon volume and operative mortality in the United States. *N Engl J Med* 2003; **349**: 2117–27.

18. Kahn JM, Goss CH, Heagerty PJ, *et al*. Hospital volume and the outcomes of mechanical ventilation. *N Engl J Med* 2006; **355**: 41–50.

19. Pearse RM, Dana EC, Lanigan CJ, Pook JAR. Organisational failures in urgent and emergency surgery. *Anaesthesia* 2001; **56**: 684–9.

20. Dyer C. Hospital trust prosecuted for not supervising junior doctors. *BMJ*. 2006; **332**: 135.

21. NCEPOD. *An acute problem?* London: NCEPOD, 2005. www.ncepod.org.uk

22. NCEPOD. *Changing the way we operate*. The 2001 report of the National Confidential Enquiry into Perioperative Deaths. London: NCEPOD, 2001. www.ncepod.org.uk

23. Fletcher SN, Kennedy DD, Ghosh IR, *et al*. Persistent neuromuscular and neurophysiologic abnormalities in long-term survivors of prolonged critical illness. *Crit Care Med* 2003; **31**: 1012–16.

24. Gordon SM, Jackson JC, Ely EW, Burger C, Hopkins RO. Clinical identification of cognitive impairment in ICU survivors: insights for intensivists. *Intens Care Med*. 2004; **30**: 1997–2008.

25. Dowdy DW, Eid MP, Sedrakyan A, *et al*. Quality of life in adult survivors of critical illness: A systematic review of the literature. *Intens Care Med* 2005; **31**: 611–20.

26. General Medical Council. *Good Medical Practice*. London: GMC, 2006. www.gmc-uk.org

27. Meiler SE. Long-term outcome after anaesthesia and surgery: remarks on the biology of a newly emerging principle in perioperative care. *Anesthesiology Clin N America* 2006; **24**: 255–78.

28. Podgoreanu MV, Schwinn DA. New paradigms in cardiovascular medicine: emerging technologies and practice – perioperative genomics. *J Am Coll Cardiol* 2005; **46**: 1965–77.

CHAPTER 6

Shamim Umarji and Martin Bircher

Pelvic and acetabular trauma

Pelvic and acetabular fractures remain a challenge for all those involved in their assessment and management. Pelvic injuries account for 3% of all musculoskeletal trauma and occur in 4–18% of those sustaining high-energy trauma[1,2,3,4] such as motor vehicle accidents and falls from heights. Males are twice as likely to be affected as females.[5] Road traffic accidents account for 73% of pelvic fractures.[5,6,7] Mortality rates in patients with pelvic fractures have been reported to range from 9 to 27%.[5] However, improved early care has resulted in a reduction of morbidity as well as mortality.[8]

It is important to note that there are significant differences between pelvic and acetabular fractures, the most notable being that the former can be associated with major haemorrhage, depending on the fracture pattern. Acetabular fractures will only rarely be associated with significant bleeding. Furthermore acetabular fractures will be associated with late post-traumatic arthritis if there is major primary articular surface loss or if the fracture remains poorly reduced after treatment. Thus delays in referral to an appropriate centre that specialises in the treatment of pelvic and pelvic–acetabular fractures will allow callus formation that hinders the possibility of complete surgical reduction of the fracture. Pelvic fractures on the other hand are often associated with gross haemodynamic and skeletal instability. The type of pelvic fracture is strongly related to the mechanism of injury, thus the taking of an accurate history is extremely important. Pelvic injuries frequently occur in areas remote from pelvic fracture reconstruction centres and this can add further logistical difficulty to their management. Within the United Kingdom the limited resources available

Recent Advances in Anaesthesia and Intensive Care 24, ed. J. N. Cashman and R. M. Grounds. Published by Cambridge University Press. © Cambridge University Press 2007.

for management of trauma and in particular with respect to pelvic and acetabular surgery, contributes to delays in definitive surgical reconstruction.[9]

Anatomy and biomechanics

The ilium, ischium, pubis and sacrum form the pelvic ring. The pelvis transmits load from the axial skeleton to the lower limbs, enabling walking. Posteriorly, stability is provided by the iliolumbar ligament, sacroiliac joint and ligaments (interosseous, anterior and posterior), the sacrospinous ligament and the sacrotuberous ligament. Anteriorly, stability is afforded by the obturator membrane complex and symphysis pubis.

The opposed bony surfaces of the pubic symphysis are covered by hyaline cartilage and united by fibrocartilage and fibrous tissue. Dense ligamentous fibres blend with the fibrocartilage anteriorly and superiorly. Inferiorly the symphysis is reinforced by the inferior pubic or arcuate ligament. Anterior stability is also provided by other soft-tissue structures such as the ilioinguinal ligament and the obturator foramen membrane.[10] The pelvic floor is composed of the muscles, ligaments, tendons and fascial planes that attach circumferentially to the pelvic outlet (Fig. 6.1). If the integrity of the pelvic floor is compromised then blood leaks in large volumes into the retroperitoneal space, often going as high as the chest as well as into the thighs (and the scrotum in males). The volume of the true pelvis is only one and a half litres and of itself does not account for the large volume of blood loss in these injuries. This observation is supported by a study into the volume changes within the disrupted pelvis.[11] It is estimated that a displaced fracture that causes symphyseal widening of 10 cm and opens the sacroiliac joint by 3 cm, will result in a mere 55% increase in true pelvic volume.[11]

Bleeding in patients with pelvic fractures that becomes a problem is usually venous rather than arterial. The pelvic veins form a massive thin-walled venous plexus through which arteries intertwine. Most drain into the internal iliac vein but some drain to the superior rectal vein then into the inferior mesenteric vein and on to the portal vein. Massive haemorrhage may arise from this venous plexus following trauma. However, the potential for arterial bleeding should not be forgotten and consideration should always be made towards exclusion of arterial bleeding, and angiography may be of use to help exclude this. Damage to nerves is also a very important by-product of pelvic fractures. The sciatic nerve leaves the pelvis between the piriformis and obturator internus through the greater sciatic notch. Other nerves at risk are the femoral, obturator, pudendal and superior gluteal nerves. All may be damaged during the injury causing the pelvic

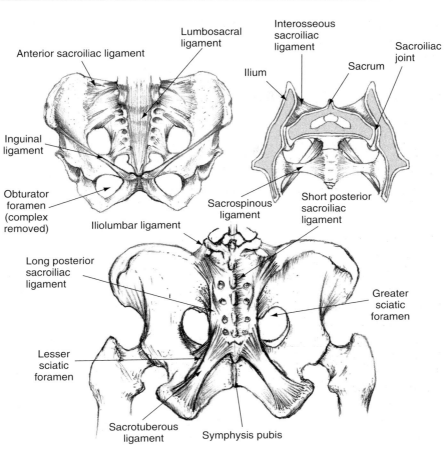

Fig. 6.1 Diagram of pelvis with key ligaments.

fracture and may be further damaged during or consequent upon the treatment required to repair the fracture. Careful assessment of the history and nature of the injury should be made and recorded and particular care should be made of examination of the x-rays of the fracture, with careful attention to the local anatomy around the fracture site(s) and consideration of the potential for nerve damage and long-term sequelae.

Patient retrieval

Ideally a patient with severe pelvic trauma should be transported rapidly to a major trauma centre with appropriate facilities for assessment and care of the patient and for appropriate pelvic surgery. However, the reality is that most patients are initially retrieved to a hospital with trauma facilities close to the scene of the accident and then subsequently referred on to a more specialist centre with facilities and expertise for definitive pelvic fracture

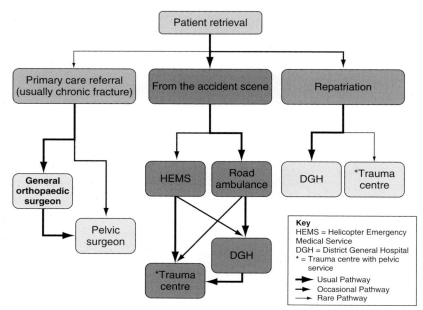

Fig 6.2 Patient retrieval.

reconstruction. Care of the patient with pelvic trauma therefore falls into two broad areas of treatment. The first phase is the immediate treatment of the patient, with stabilisation of the fracture and treatment of any other life-threatening injuries. The second phase is the definitive treatment of the pelvic or acetabular fracture. Thus a patient can be triaged in a number of different ways as shown in the flow chart in Fig. 6.2.

Patient evaluation in the resuscitation room

In the resuscitation room when the patient is initially assessed at the scene of the accident or in the trauma room of the hospital to which they are first taken, the assessment of these patients using an ATLS (Advance Trauma Life Support) approach is mandatory. The decision-making should address the need for life-saving surgery (either immediate or within the first 24 hours), damage control surgery and early total or delayed definitive surgery. The decision should be based on clinical criteria such as haemo-dynamic status, physiological criteria (hypothermia, acidosis and coagulo-pathy) and scoring of injury severity. The primary aim is to ensure control of the airway and any damage to the respiratory system; to control and stop any bleeding; and to provide cardiovascular and respiratory stability. The term damage control was popularised by Rotondo in 1993 for the successful treatment of penetrating abdominal injuries.[12] Following this approach surgery may also include rapid abbreviate laparotomy to stop haemorrhage and peritoneal contamination, and staged sequential repair after ongoing resuscitation. It is this term by Rotondo that has led to the principle of 'damage control orthopaedics'.[13] The philosophy here is one of early stabilisation of long-bone fractures which, when extended to pelvic injuries, means abbreviated surgical procedures to control haemorrhage (external fixation), debridement and, in the case of associated damage to bowel, particularly in the case of pelvic fractures, the diversion of faeces to ensure that the fracture site is kept clean. This reduces the mortality rate and the incidence of complications.[14] Thus if there is any doubt as to the integrity of the bowel, particularly the large bowel, then early fashioning of a defunctioning colostomy proximal to the damaged bowel site will help to ensure that the fracture site in the pelvis is not contaminated with faecal flora and may be life saving. Similarly consideration should also be made as to the integrity of the urinary tract. Bladder damage and urethral damage are common in patients with fractures of the pelvis, and in patients with severe pelvis fractures a high index of suspicion as to the possibility of bladder or bowel injury should be part of the initial assessment.

Regardless of whether the patient will be definitively treated at the hospital to which he has presented or transferred to a tertiary referral centre, a primary survey and resuscitation is the starting point. Patients can only be transferred to tertiary centres once physiologically stable.

Primary survey

As for any trauma patient, the ATLS Guidelines (Committee on Trauma. American College of Surgeons) must take precedence and guide initial assessment and resuscitation. Thus, the patient should be triaged in such a way as to sequence the priorities of emergency medical care, and undergo a primary and secondary evaluation to ensure this sequence of priorities is correct. This should start with the essential ABCDE of trauma care.

A: Control of the airway with cervical spine control
B: Breathing and ventilation
C: Circulation with haemorrhage control
D: Disability/neurological status
E: Exposure (assessment or evaluation) of all injuries

The expected blood loss in patients with pelvic fractures can be estimated from the extent of injuries. Major haemorrhage is associated with antero-posterior and vertical shear-type fractures[15] with large-volume blood loss from the venous plexus and branches of the iliac veins and fractured bony surface. Major arterial disruption is not usually survivable. Arterial bleeding with pelvic fractures is usually from smaller vessels, e.g. superior gluteal, obturator and pudendal arteries. The Burgess and Young[15] classification of pelvic fractures links the type of pelvic fracture with blood loss. In the broadest terms fractures that crumple the pelvic floor bleed less than those that tear it. Certain pelvic fracture patterns bleed more than others, depending on the mechanism. Focused assessment for sonographic examination of the trauma patient (FAST) may assist in this primary survey. It is worth remembering that 40% of patients with pelvic fractures have an intra-abdominal source of bleeding (liver, spleen, bowel, bladder/urinary tract).

In the resuscitation phase, shock management should be initiated if appropriate. Management of patient oxygenation is continuously reassessed and haemorrhage control is repeatedly re-evaluated. Large-bore venous access is achieved. Replacement of lost vascular volume with warmed crystalloids may be started, as are other modalities of shock therapy where appropriate. Control of the airway and management of respiration is ensured. Tissue aerobic metabolism is assured by ensuring tissue perfusion with well-oxygenated red blood cells. Arterial blood gas analysis, haematocrit, haemoglobin, lactate level, base deficit, pH, blood type, cross match and clotting are performed urgently. Fluid resuscitation depends on the patient's response to an initial volume load (2 L of pre-warmed crystalloids). The 'responder' may require no more than the initial crystalloid given. The 'transient responder' may need typed and cross-matched blood. It may be appropriate to place a urinary catheter and a nasogastric tube during this phase if its use is not contraindicated. The administration of platelets, fresh frozen plasma (FFP) or fibrinogen is well established in patients with unstable pelvic fractures. Hypotensive patients (systolic BP < 90 mmHg) with 'transient response' to resuscitation should undergo urgent surgery for damage-control procedures. The non-responders need life-saving surgical treatment and all patients must be kept warm. There are physiological criteria which can aid the decision to initiate damage-control surgery. The 'Lethal Triad'[13] comprises hypothermia ($< 34\,°C$), coagulopathy (prothrombin time > 19s or platelet count $< 90\,000$) and acidosis (pH < 7.2 or lactate $> 5\,\mathrm{mmol.l^{-1}}$)

Patients with pelvic or pelvic–acetabular fractures can be categorised as follows:

- Stable fracture/stable patient

- Stable fracture/unstable patient (consider other source of haemorrhage, e.g. abdomen)

- Unstable fracture/stable patient ('responder')

- Unstable fracture/unstable patient (transient or 'non-responder')

Once the primary survey has been completed according to ATLS protocol, then efforts should be focused on preventing further loss of blood.

Steps to control pelvic bleeding associated with pelvic fractures

Control of blood loss will depend on availability of time, the institution and its resources and available expertise. In other words not all institutions have, for example, the availability of pelvic external fixators or surgeons with the skill to apply them. Nonetheless, the following are some methods to control pelvic bleeding including, when appropriate, emergency surgery such as laparotomy.

Pelvic binding: Unnecessary movement of the patient should be avoided. Pelvic binders can be helpful (in the absence of a proprietary binder an emergency one can be made by wrapping a sheet around the pelvis and pulling this tight to close the open pelvic fracture. This will close the potential space of the pelvis and may tamponade the blood loss long enough for the team to get control over the bleeding) and the legs should be wrapped together (internal rotation and adduction of lower limbs). This will partially reduce the fracture.

External fixation: External fixator devices are used in some centres for haemodynamically unstable patients with severe pelvic ring disruption.

Packing: Emergency laparotomy and packing in conjunction with external fixation may be necessary and should be considered in the patient with severe bleeding that is not rapidly diminishing and is of unknown origin.

Internal fixation: Urgent open reduction and internal fixation of the pelvic fracture may be performed in appropriate situations when there are suitably experienced pelvic orthopaedic surgeons available.

Embolisation: Arterial and venous embolisation under x-ray control performed in the radiology department may also be considered. This is usually reserved for modest bleeding – for example, a patient requiring 2–3 units of blood every 24 hours. The use of embolisation is controversial and is very institution dependent. Not all institutions can offer this service on a 24-hour basis owing to insufficient numbers of appropriately trained radiologists. If embolisation is available on a 24-hour basis then this mode of haemorrhage control is more likely to be used earlier in the resuscitation process.

Use of external fixation

The role and use of external fixator devices in the acute setting remain controversial. Reimer[16] has shown a reduction in mortality through the use of external fixators, though this has not been reproduced elsewhere. The role of the external fixator will depend on the individual surgeon and the particular case scenario.

Indications for the use of an external pelvic fixator include:

- Emergency – for stabilisation of fractures to aid resuscitation and aid blood loss
- Temporary – prior to definitive fixation
- Definitive – for management of some fractures (antero-posterior compression)
- Supplementary – to augment definitive surgery and, in reverse, for lateral compression

Once the primary survey has been completed and immediate life-threatening haemorrhage has been contained then it is important to proceed to complete a secondary survey.

Secondary survey

The secondary survey does not begin until the primary survey has been completed and the resuscitation phase (management of life-threatening conditions) has begun. Potential spinal fracture precautions are maintained until the spine is clinically and radiologically cleared. Evaluation and treatment must occur simultaneously. The secondary survey is a 'head-to-toe' evaluation which involves in-depth evaluation, including a thorough history and examination. Details of the accident from the paramedics are essential. This provides clues as to the nature of the pelvic injury sustained. For example, a man falling 6 feet (2 metres) off a ladder on to his side is likely to sustain an anterior column acetabular fracture, whereas a patient falling from the fourth floor is more likely to have a major pelvic disruption with significant soft-tissue damage. Other concomitant medical conditions, allergies and last meal intake should be elicited in the history. Each region of the body must be individually assessed and examined. It is vital at this stage that a full neurological assessment is made. Many patients with pelvic fractures suffer from neurological damage associated with the pelvic fracture and it is vital that full evaluation of the damage is made at as early a stage as possible and that any definitive treatment is started as soon as possible.

Definitive care phase

In the definitive care phase, all the patient's injuries are managed. This phase includes comprehensive management, fracture stabilisation, any required operative intervention and transfer if appropriate to a specialist pelvic fracture reconstruction centre.

Treat or transfer

The decision to treat or transfer will depend on a number of different factors including experience of staff, size of hospital, and whether or not the orthopaedic team is experienced in the management of pelvic and pelvic acetabular fractures. In most cases the patient will require transfer to a specialist unit for further definitive management.[9] Once the patient is stable from the cardiorespiratory point of view this no longer assumes the same urgency as the initial resuscitation when the patient was first admitted to the hospital from the scene of the accident. After haemodynamic stabilisation of the patient, if definitive reconstruction is necessary, then a decision to transfer should be made rapidly. Patients should undergo reconstructive surgery within five days of the initial injury, if this is possible.[9] However, caution must be observed in the transfer of the patient between hospitals. Patients should not be transferred where the risk of the transfer is sufficiently great that it will exacerbate any other injury. This is of particular importance with respect to patients with chest injuries and lung contusions. Thus patients with lung contusion who are receiving artificial ventilation in an intensive care unit (ICU) should not be transferred in the early stages for a number of reasons. If they are stable then their chest contusion will improve more rapidly if they are not moved. Transport of ventilated patients between two hospital sites has been shown consistently to be detrimental. Part of the reason for this is that the transport ventilators in ambulances are simply not as sophisticated as the modern ICU ventilator. Another reason for deterioration in this situation may be the fact that the patient has to be moved from bed to trolley to ambulance back to trolley and back to the bed in the receiving hospital. All of these moves contribute to the deterioration that is frequently seen when these very sick patients with complex lung problems caused by traumatic contusions are moved between hospitals. Furthermore the move may be counterproductive because if the patient's lung condition is sufficiently severe to warrant artificial ventilation in ICU then the patient is not in a state to undergo semi-elective surgery to repair the pelvic fracture, particularly if the pelvic fracture is large and the surgery is likely to take 4–6 hours with a blood loss of greater than 2.5 litres. Definitive surgery should be postponed until the patient's cardiovascular and respiratory systems and physiology are sufficiently stable to undertake a safe inter-hospital transfer, and then when they arrive at the receiving hospital to be able to undergo the definitive surgery for the reconstruction of the pelvic fractures.

Indications for and timing of pelvic and acetabular fracture surgery

Ideally surgery should be performed as soon as safely possible but this will be governed by patient factors (haemodynamic and immunological status) and resource factors (hospital type, surgical expertise). The 'second hit' phenomenon needs to be avoided.[13] Damage-control surgery entails performing the least invasive surgical procedure that preserves life and prevents death by exsanguination whilst reducing the risk of multiorgan failure (MOF), systemic inflammatory response (SIRS) and acute respiratory distress syndrome (ARDS).

Indications for urgent pelvic and acetabular fracture surgery

The indications for immediate (day 0) pelvic surgery are outlined in Fig. 6.3, whilst the indications for urgent acetabular surgery are outlined in Tables 6.1a and 6.1b.

Reconstruction of pelvic and acetabular fractures

As already stated, definitive surgery should be performed as soon as patient and resource factors allow. The patient must be haemodynamically and immunologically stable. Only when parameters such as the haemodynamic state, blood gas analysis, serum lactate, base deficit and urine output have stabilised, can surgery be safely performed. If patients are not already in a centre that is able to undertake definitive acetabular reconstruction then they should be transferred to such a centre as soon as possible. This should ideally take place within a few days of the initial injury with the aim of

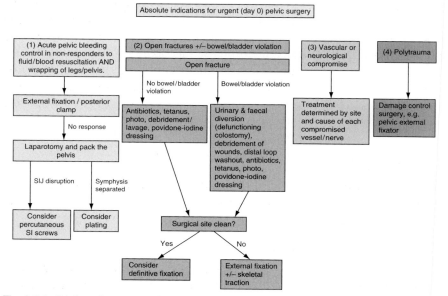

Fig. 6.3 Indications for urgent pelvic surgery; SI = Sacroiliac; SIJ = Sacroiliac joint.

Table 6.1a Indications for urgent acetabular reconstruction.

Open fractures
Worsening neurological status
Vascular compromise
Irreducible fracture dislocation
As part of an acute pelvic fixation

Table 6.1b Other indications for acetabular reconstruction.

Acetabular fractures with urological injury
Hip instability (recurrent dislocation) despite traction
Acetabular fracture with ipsilateral femoral fracture

undertaking the reconstruction within two to five days of the initial injury. In countries where there is a well-developed trauma service this is the usual practice. In the United Kingdom, where trauma services are not as well developed, the delay in undertaking is often as long as ten days with the consequent increase in long-term complications.[9]

Operative management

Emergency surgery

The principles of management are adequate resuscitation first. Surgery should be kept short and to a minimum and this will be primarily determined by the surgeon. Good communications between anaesthetist and the surgeon are essential. Technical aspects include careful monitoring of urine output, arterial blood gas analysis (serum lactate, pH, base excess), and central venous pressure. During the time in theatre the patient should be kept well hydrated and warm. Finally, the team must be aware of their limitations and when it is appropriate to safely curtail surgery for the best overall outcome.

Elective surgery

It helps to divide procedures into small, medium and large pelvic and acetabular operations. This enables appropriate patient preparation before, during and after surgery.

Operative-size classification

There is great variation in what comprises a pelvic or acetabular fracture. Some fractures have a much greater impact because of their multifragmentary and highly displaced nature, which makes the proposed surgery a totally different prospect to a fracture that is simple (i.e. not multifragmentary) and minimally displaced. It is therefore helpful for surgeons, anaesthetists and all theatre personnel to classify fractures into 'small', 'medium' and 'large' (Table 6.2).

'Small' fractures: Examples of 'small' fracture procedures are external fixator only, pubic symphysis plating, percutaneous fixation, posterior wall fixation (Kocher–Langenbach approach with patient positioned lateral or prone). Such procedures are likely to require 4 units of cross-matched blood and two large-bore IV cannulae. The use of red cell saver is advisable.

'Medium' fractures: Examples of 'medium' pelvic and acetabular procedures are symphysis pubis plating and percutaneous posterior screws (patient supine), anterior acetabular fracture fixation through the Stoppa approach (patient supine), internal fixation of transverse/posterior wall acetabular fracture via a Kocher–Langenbach approach (the patient is positioned laterally or prone depending on the surgeon's preference). For these procedures 6 units of cross-matched blood, two large-bore IV cannulae, a CVP line and red cell saver are advisable.

'Large' fractures: Examples of 'large' fracture procedures are 'front and back' open pelvic surgery such as a posterior plating of iliac fracture (patient prone) and anterior column acetabular fracture fixation (patient supine). Ilioinguinal approaches for acetabular fractures, where most of the fracture is anterior (patient supine) and double approaches to acetabulum, e.g. both column fractures (patient supine and prone) are also large procedures. For these fractures 8 units of cross-matched blood, a CVP line, red cell saver, arterial line monitoring and the patient admitted to the critical care unit (ICU or HDU) postoperatively are all advised.

Modifiers of operative-size classification

Using this simple classification system in certain circumstances fractures can be up- or downgraded. Combined acetabular and pelvic surgery is automatically placed into the 'large' group. The operation should be moved up to the next group if the patient has serious concomitant injuries to other parts of the body. If injuries are more than two weeks old, then these are reclassified into a higher group. If other procedures are performed at the same time, then again the fracture is reclassified into a higher group. Finally, if the patient is already in the 'large' group and needs to be classified up a level, then a suffix of ' + ' may be added. This would be the highest level.

The single most important concomitant injury is to the chest and lung parenchyma. Many patients with fractures of the pelvis suffered as a

Table 6.2 Summary of operative size and suggested requirements.

Size of operation	Examples	Blood cross-match	Vascular access/special requirements	Likely blood loss	Operative time
Small	– Posterior wall fracture – Isolated symphysis pubis diastasis – Isolated iliac crescent fracture	4 units	2x IV cannulae Urinary catheter	<1L	<2 hrs
Medium	– Posterior column fracture – Anterior column fracture – Anterior wall fracture – Anterior pelvic fixation and percutaneous posterior fixation – External fixation and open posterior pelvic surgery	6 units	2x IV cannulae Cell saver Urinary catheter +/– CVP line +/– Arterial line +/– HDU bed	1–2 L	2–4 hrs
Large	– Open anterior and posterior pelvic surgery – 'T'-shaped acetabular fracture – Associated both column fracture (ABC) – Anterior column and posterior hemi-transverse fracture	8 units	2x IV cannulae CVP line Arterial line Cell saver, urinary catheter, HDU/ITU bed	2–5 L	4–6 hrs

consequence of motor vehicle accidents also suffer injuries to the chest and chest wall. These must always be taken seriously, even if on initial investigation they seem quite minor. The consequences of a high-energy impact that is sufficient to fracture one or more ribs will inevitably cause significant blunt trauma to the underlying lung. Surgery and anaesthesia for a prolonged operation to repair and reconstruct the pelvic fracture will inevitably cause a large cytokine release and there is a very great chance that by the end of the surgery or in the immediate postoperative period what had been perceived as only minor chest trauma prior to the start of surgery will have developed into full-blown ARDS with the well-known consequences of the two conditions. To avoid this, surgery should be postponed until the lung injury is healed or at the very least has settled. Anaesthetists should be aware of the potential complication and should be alert to deteriorating lung function during the course of major surgery in patients who suffered what initially appeared to be minor lung contusions. Anaesthetists should also be aware that 'large' operations will inevitably result in large intraoperative blood loss. Blood loss for these cases will be 2–5 litres and the anaesthetic technique should reflect this potential for massive haemorrhage. Patients should be prepared with sufficient intravenous access to cope with a blood loss of greater than 2.5 litres.

Other anaesthetic considerations

Regional anaesthesia is not appropriate. It is very difficult, if not impossible, to perform a regional block in a patient with a fractured pelvis. The patient is unable to sit up because of the pain and the patient is unable to turn on his/her side or curl up sufficiently to perform epidural anaesthesia. Furthermore if the patient already has some form of pelvic fracture external fixator device or skeletal traction then it is impossible to perform epidural analgesia prior to the commencement of surgery. Many patients will already have nerve damage from the original accident. Finally, there is a very high likelihood that postoperatively there may be nerve damage caused by the surgery, as well as the potential for compartment syndrome. It is thus vital that the surgeons are able to assess the patient's neurology and the limb viability immediately after the end of the surgery. This cannot be satisfactorily achieved in the presence of a regional block, which may mask the symptoms and signs of these two potentially catastrophic complications.

All patients will require general anaesthesia. Most patients undergoing these operations are young and, being fit and healthy prior to surgery (most being victims of motor vehicle accidents), they will tolerate quite large doses of opioid for their intra-and postoperative analgesic requirements. It is not uncommon to require 30–40 mg morphine intra-operatively and a further 30–100 mg intravenous morphine in the immediate 12–24 hours postoperatively. All patients will require measures to ensure that heat loss is kept to a minimum, with warming blankets and thorough warming of all intravenous fluids. Temperature measurements should be made. The use of a red-cell salvage technique is recommended.

Open fractures

Open pelvic fractures account for 2–4% of all pelvic injuries.[2,17,18,19,20] Such fractures are considered open if they communicate with the external environment or if there is a concomitant bowel perforation resulting in potential or actual faecal contamination. Open injuries are associated with high-energy impact commonly involving motor vehicles. Some reports place open pelvic fractures with wounds extending into the perineum or rectum automatically into the Gustilo and Anderson type-3 injury category.[2] Bircher[21] classifies open fractures into three basic types, as shown in Table 6.3.

Closed internal degloving injuries (Morel–Lavallee lesion) occur in up to 16% of patients.[22] This is the result of soft-tissue stripping off the fascia, and haematoma formation. The resultant fat necrosis and ischaemic skin flaps lead to bacterial colonisation as high as 46%.[22] Such lesions should be debrided before, during and after surgery. The degloved area is generally left open and allowed to heal by secondary intention. These areas may also need the assistance of the plastic surgery teams at the time of surgery, making the surgery much more complex and lasting longer. This should be taken into consideration when the anaesthesia team is planning for the surgery. Open fractures will inevitably make the patients postoperative course much more complicated. These patients will often spend prolonged periods of time in the intensive care unit and may require frequent return to the operating theatre for debridement and washout of the infected region. If the bone becomes infected from the contamination either by bowel contents or from the original open wound then the results can be disastrous and all efforts must be made to ensure that open fractures do not progress to osteomyelitis of the pelvic bones.

Table 6.3 Classification of open fractures.

A Type	'Outside in'
B Type	'Inside out'
C Type	Severe soft-tissue injury or faecal contamination

Associated injuries

Urogenital injury

Rupture of the bladder and urethra occurs in up to 20% of patients with a fractured pelvis and pubic rami fractures (particularly from straddle injuries). Urethral injuries occur in up to 15% of men but are rare in women. In males the supramembranous portion of the urethra (bulbous urethra) is the most common site of injury. Injury may also occur in the cavernous and or prostatic portion of the urethra. Indications of urethral injury include blood at the meatus, a high-riding prostate at rectal examination and a straddle-type fracture of the pelvic ring. Urogenital injury is promptly diagnosed by a urethrocystogram performed in the resuscitation room. Drainage of urine as soon as possible is important. Bladder and urethral injuries occur in up to 21% of cases.[7] They can often be predicted from the fracture pattern. Radiographic features such as widening of the sacroiliac joint, pubic symphysis diastasis and sacral fractures are associated with bladder injury. Patients with displaced rami fractures and sacroiliac joint disruptions may be at especially high risk of urogenital injury and consideration should be made to performing initial retrograde urethrograms before attempting instrumentation of the urethra.

Bladder rupture requires prompt diagnosis, so as to avoid hyperkalaemia, hypernatraemia, uraemia, acidosis and peritonitis. The rupture may be extraperitoneal or intraperitoneal (or both). If it is extraperitoneal the rupture is most commonly anterior, but rarely may result from laceration from a sharp bone spike. In many case this can be treated non-operatively with suprapubic drainage. Intraperitoneal rupture occurs in about 15% of major pelvic fractures, most often from contusion to the lower abdomen or the sympyseal region. It may also occur in association with pelvic ring disruptions as the result of seatbelt injuries or steering wheel injury.

A high incidence of pelvic floor dysfunction in a study of 24 consecutive women has been noted. Sixteen women had de novo pelvic floor dysfunction, 12 had bladder symptoms and seven out of the 17 sexually active women had sexual dysfunction.[23] The incidence of sexual dysfunction rises to 42% when there is an associated urological injury. The incidence of erectile dysfunction is 12% and dyspareunia 2% when considering all high-energy pelvic fractures.[24] It is vital therefore if there is any urogenital injury or even suspicion of injury that the urologists are involved in the care of the patient from a very early stage, preferably at the time of admission with the initial injury.

Anorectal injury

Anorectal injuries have an incidence of between 1 and 2% when associated with a pelvic fracture.[17,19] They may include lacerations of the rectum, and perforations of small or large bowel. Often tears will be accompanied by perineal wounds. There is a much higher incidence with open pelvic fractures, with anorectal injuries occurring in up to 64%.[25] A rectal examination in the secondary survey is mandatory to exclude anorectal injury. The clinician examines for blood in the rectum or palpable bony fragments, which would lead one to suspect bowel perforation. These are considered to be open fractures and as such require urgent surgery in the form of laparotomy and faecal diversion (i.e. a colostomy). The team leader at the time of the secondary survey in the ATLS protocol may not be the orthopaedic surgeon and it is vital that the team leader understands the potential for future problems and ensures that the general surgeons are involved, and arranges for appropriate faecal diversion in these cases. Delay in obtaining faecal diversion and washout of the affected stump of colon will increase the likelihood of future complications and death. The main concern is faecal contamination of the fracture site resulting in overwhelming sepsis and death. Perineal injury incurs a high incidence (77%) of sepsis.[20]

Neurological injury

The sciatic nerve is particularly vulnerable after acetabular fractures associated with posterior dislocation of the hip. It is therefore essential to examine specifically for this during the secondary survey. The mechanism of injury is either direct neural injury from a sacral fracture or indirect injury from traction accompanying the pelvic displacement. Injury to the lumbosacral plexus is common, with L5 and S1 roots being the most likely to be damaged. Careful documentation of the presence of a complete or partial foot drop with any associated numbness is important for clinical as well as medicolegal reasons. Neurological injury may occur at the time of injury or may develop postoperatively, hence the importance of careful documentation. The incidence of sciatic nerve palsy is 12% according to Letournel and Judets series of 940 patients.[26] Femoral head dislocation occurs in 32–39% of acetabular fractures.[8,27] Recovery of the nerve is variable. In contrast femoral nerve injury is rare and recovery on the whole more likely.

A CT scan can be useful in determining the exact morphology of sacral fractures especially when they involve the sacral canal. Sacral fractures have been classified by Denis[28] into those lateral to the foramina (zone 1), transforaminal (zone 2), and those medial to the foramina extending into

the sacral canal (zone 3). The latter are associated with the greatest incidence of nerve injury, with the cauda equina being at most risk. The L5
nerve root is vulnerable in zone 1 injuries, and unilateral sacral nerve roots
in zone 2.

Outcomes

Improvements in the management of high-energy trauma over recent decades has resulted in a decline in mortality rates. According to a German
multicentre study, pelvic injury was the main cause of death in only 0.9% of
cases.[29] Mortality rises to 25–30% for open fractures.[30,31] Factors affecting
mortality include age (the adult population being worse affected than the
paediatric population), hypotension on arrival at the resuscitation room
(highlighting patients as either transient or non-responders), pelvic instability (and hence a greater degree of vascular instability), extent of wound
(large soft-tissue trauma, degloving, open and Morel–Lavellee injuries),
presence of rectal injury, whether a blood transfusion is required and
associated injuries.[17,19] The overall improvement in mortality rates can
be attributed to a better understanding of the natural history of these
patients. Targeted care on presentation to the resuscitation room, improved
critical care facilities and an early multidisciplinary approach, including
aggressive fracture stabilisation and the practise of urinary/faecal diversion
in the case of open pelvic fractures, have all contributed to better overall
outcome.

The morbidity associated with these injuries is significant not only in the
short term, but also in the long term. Patients can develop chronic problems
which have a serious impact on their working lives. The sequelae and
complications of the injury and the resulting investigations and surgery
can be divided into immediate, early and late (Table 6.4).

Conclusion

Pelvic and acetabular fractures usually occur in high-energy impacts and as
such frequently arise in polytrauma and other potentially life-threatening
injuries. An early 'total care' approach is required for such patients, with
important input from the anaesthetic and critical care teams throughout.
When faced with such patients in the acute setting, ATLS and 'damage
control orthopaedic' principles are utilised. The 'early treatment phase'
comprises haemorrhage control (pelvic external fixator, pelvic packing),
soft-tissue debridement, faecal diversion (defunctioning colostomy) and
treatment of urogenital injury. The 'definitive treatment phase' comprises
anatomical fracture stabilisation and definitive soft-tissue management.

Table 6.4 Complications which are usually associated with either or both pelvic and acetabular fractures.

	Immediate	Early	Late
Pelvic (P)	Haemorrhage – anteroposterior compression and vertical shear injuries have a higher incidence of pelvic vascular injury, massive transfusion, systemic inflammatory response syndrome, urethral disruption, bladder rupture, rectal perforation, vaginal wall laceration	Transfusion-related acute lung injury, acute respiratory distress syndrome, multiorgan dysfunction syndrome, coagulopathy resulting in thromboembolic events, e.g. thrombosis pulmonary embolus, disseminated intravascular coagulation	Chronic pelvic pain, pelvic asymmetry leading to chronic pain, erectile dysfunction, urethral stricture
Acetabular (A)	Hip dislocation/subluxation	Hip dislocation/subluxation	Post-traumatic osteoarthritis, AVN of femoral head, leg length discrepancy
Both (P and A)	Emboli (thrombus, fat, air), sciatic, sacral plexus, femoral and obturator nerve injuries	Nerve palsies, septicaemia, wound infection, deep infection, haematoma	Trendelenberg gait, inability to return to work for prolonged period, psychosocial problems, e.g. post-traumatic stress disorder, growth arrest in paediatric fractures

AVN: avascular necrosis.

Management of such patients requires a team approach and as such good communication between staff, especially surgeon and anaesthetist, is essential. In an attempt to 'speak the same language' pelvic and acetabular fractures can be classified into 'small', 'medium' and 'large', which aids the anaesthetist as well as other theatre staff when definitive reconstruction is undertaken.

References

1. Inaba K, Sharkey PW, Stephen DJ. The increasing incidence of pelvic ring injury in motor vehicle collisions. *Injury* 2004; **35**: 759–65.
2. Groltz MR, Allami K, Harwood P, *et al*. Open pelvic fractures: epidemiology, current concepts of management and outcome. *Injury* 2005; **36**: 1–13.
3. Clancy TV, Gary MJ, Covington DL. A state-wide analysis of level 1 and 2 trauma centres for patients with major injuries. *J Trauma* 2001; **51**: 346–51.
4. Muir L, Boot D, Gorman DF. The epidemiology of pelvic fractures in the Mersey region. *Injury* 1996; **27**: 199–204.
5. Gansslen A, Pohlmann T, Paul C. Epidemiology of pelvic ring injuries. *Injury* 1996; 27(Suppl 1); S20.
6. Poole GV, Ward EF. Causes of mortality in patients with pelvic fractures. *Orthopaedics* 1994; **17**: 691–6.
7. Rommens PM, Hessmann MH. Staged reconstruction of pelvic ring disruption: differences in morbidity, mortality, radiologic results and functional outcomes between B1, B2/B3, C-type lesions. *J Orthop Trauma* 2002; **16**: 92–8.
8. Matta JM. Fractures of the acetabulum: accuracy of reduction and clinical results in patients managed operatively within 3 weeks after injury. *J Bone Joint Surg Am* 1996; **78**: 1632–45.
9. Madhu R, Kotnis R, Willett K, *et al*. Outcome of surgery for reconstruction of fractures of the acetabulum. Time dependent effects of delay. *J Bone Joint Surg* 2006; **88**: 1197–203.
10. Vrahas MS, Hern TC, Diangelo D, Kellam J, Tile M. Ligamentous contributions to pelvic stability. *Orthopaedics* 1995; **18**: 271–4.
11. Moss MC, Bircher MD. Volume changes within the true pelvis during disruption of the pelvic ring – where does the haemorrhage go? *Injury* 1996; **27** (Suppl 1): SA21–3.
12. Rotondo MF, Schwab W. "Damage Control": an approach for improved survival in exsanguinating penetrating abdominal injury. *J Trauma* 1993; **35**: 375–82.
13. Pape H-C, Giannoudis P, Krettek C. Timing of fixation of major fractures in blunt polytrauma: role of conventional indicators in clinical decision making. *J Orthop Trauma* 2005; **19**: 551–623.
14. Ertel W, Keel M, Eid K. Control of severe haemorrhage using C clamp and pelvic packing in multiply injured patients with pelvic ring disruption. *J Orthop Trauma* 2001; **15**: 468–74.
15. Burgess AR, Eastridge BJ, Young JW, *et al*. Pelvic ring disruptions: effective classification system and treatment protocols. *J Trauma* 1990; **30**: 848–56.
16. Reimer BL, Butterfield SL, Diamond DL, Young JC. Acute mortality associated with injuries to the pelvic ring: the role of early patient mobilisation and external fixation. *J Trauma* 1993; **35**: 671–5.

17. Brennemen FD, Katyal D, Boulanger BR, Tile M. Long-term outcomes in open pelvic fractures. *J Trauma* 1997; **42**: 773–7.
18. Perry Jr. JF. Pelvic open fractures. *Clin Orthop Relat Research* 1980; 41–5.
19. Ferrera P C, Hill D A. Good outcomes in open pelvic fractures. *Injury* 1999; **30**: 187–90.
20. Jones AL, Powell J, Kellam JF, McCormack RG. Open pelvic fractures. A multicentre retrospective analysis. *Orthop Clin North Am* 1997; **28**: 345–50.
21. Bircher M, Hargrove R. Is it possible to classify open fractures of the pelvis? *Europ J Trauma* 2004; **30**: 74–91.
22. Hak DJ, Olson SA, Matta JM. Diagnosis and management of closed internal degloving injuries associated with pelvic and acetabular fractures: the Morel–Lavallee lesion. *J Trauma* 1997; **42**: 1046–51.
23. Baessler K, Bircher M, Stanton S. Pelvic floor dysfunction in women after pelvic trauma. *Br J Obstet Gynaecol* 2004; **111**: 499–502.
24. King J. Impotence after fractures of the pelvis. *J Bone Joint Surg Am* 1975; **57**: 1107–09.
25. Sinnott R, Rhodes M, Brader A. Open pelvic fracture: an injury for trauma centres. *Am J Surg* 1992; **163**: 283–7.
26. Letournel E, Judet R (eds.). *Fractures of the Acetabulum*. 2nd edn. Berlin: Springer, 1993.
27. Alonso JE, Davila R, Bradley E. Extended iliofemoral versus triradiate approaches in the management of associated acetabular fractures. *Clin Orthop Relat Res* 1994; **305**: 81–7.
28. Denis F, Davis S, Comfort T. Sacral fractures: an important problem. Retrospective analysis of 236 cases. *Clin Orthop Relat Res* 1988; **227**: 67–8.
29. Pohlemann T, Tscherne H, Baumgartel F. Pelvic fractures: epidemiology, therapy and long-term outcome. Overview of the multicentre study of the pelvis group. *Unfallchirurg* 1996; **99**: 160–7.
30. Rothenberger D, Fischer R P, Strate R. The mortality associated with pelvic fractures. *Surgery* 1978; **84**: 356–61.
31. Maull K, Sachatello CR, Ernst CB. The deep perineal laceration: an injury frequently associated with open pelvic fractures: a need for aggressive surgical management. *J Trauma* 1977; **17**: 685–96.

S. *Nicholas Fletcher*

Echocardiography

Echocardiography or cardiac ultrasound has long been established as an important cardiac imaging technique for acquiring real-time information about cardiac anatomy and function. The technological aspect of this cardiac ultrasound platform continues to evolve and also to migrate across patient populations, different specialities and clinical usage. Cardiac assessment and monitoring have always been an essential part of the management of the patient undergoing anaesthesia and intensive care. This chapter provides an overview of the more recent clinical aspects, training issues, technological advances and future developments in relation to these areas.

Clinical uses of echocardiography

Cardiac anaesthesia and cardiac critical care

The current interest in echocardiography by anaesthetists can be traced back to a group of cardiac anaesthetists in North America who adopted intra-operative transoesophageal echocardiography (TOE). To a varying extent they have displaced cardiologists from the cardiac theatre and developed practice guidelines and education programmes.[1] This approach has been widely emulated in cardiac anaesthetic practice in the UK and in parts of Europe.[2] Although no data are currently available for contemporary UK practice, 72% of anaesthetists who responded to a survey in the United States personally employed intra-operative TOE during cardiac surgery.[3] This figure was 35% in a Canadian survey.[4] In my own institution, intra-operative TOE is provided almost exclusively by anaesthetists, with over 400 intra-operative studies performed during 2005.

Recent Advances in Anaesthesia and Intensive Care 24, ed. J. N. Cashman and R. M. Grounds.
Published by Cambridge University Press. © Cambridge University Press 2007.

Table 7.1 Indications for echocardiography for cardiac surgery and intensive care.

Category I indications
Preoperative
  Unstable patients with suspected thoracic aortic aneurysms, dissection or disruption who need to be evaluated quickly

Intra-operative
  Assessment of aortic valve function in repair of aortic dissections with possible aortic valve involvement
  Evaluation of acute, persistent and life-threatening haemodynamic disturbances in which ventricular function and its determinants are uncertain and have not responded to treatment
  Evaluation of pericardial window procedures
  Congenital heart conditions (for most lesions requiring cardiopulmonary bypass)
  Patients with endocarditis in whom preoperative testing was inadequate or extension of infection to perivalvular tissue is suspected
  Repair of hypertrophic obstructive cardiomyopathy
  Valve repair

Other
  Unstable patients in ITU with unexplained haemodynamic disturbances, suspected valve disease or thromboembolic problems

Category II indications
Preoperative
  Assessment of patients with suspected acute thoracic aortic aneurysms, dissection or disruption

Intra-operative
  Assessment of valve replacement
  Assessment of repair of cardiac aneurysms
  Detection of foreign bodies
  Detection of air emboli during cardiotomy, heart transplant operations and upright neurosurgical procedures
  Detection of aortic atheromatous disease or other sources of aortic emboli
  Evaluation of removal of cardiac tumours
  Evaluation of pericardiectomy, pericardial effusions or evaluation of pericardial surgery
  Evaluation of anastomotic sites during heart and/or lung transplantation
  Intracardiac thrombectomy
  Pulmonary embolectomy
  Repair of thoracic aortic dissections without suspected aortic valve involvement
  Suspected cardiac trauma

Perioperative
  Patients with increased risk of myocardial ischaemia or infarction
  Patients with increased risk of haemodynamic disturbances

Other
  Monitoring placement and function of assist devices

Category III indications
Intra-operative
  Assessment of repair of thoracic aortic injuries
  Evaluation of myocardial perfusion, coronary anatomy or graft patency
  Evaluation of pleuropulmonary diseases
  Monitoring for emboli during orthopaedic procedures
  Repair of cardiomyopathies other than hypertrophic obstructive cardiomyopathy
  Uncomplicated endocarditis during non-cardiac surgery
  Uncomplicated pericarditis

Other
  Monitoring placement of intra-aortic balloon pumps, automatic implantable cardiac defibrillators or pulmonary artery catheters

Adapted from: Thys, D. M., Abel, M., Bollen, B. A. et al.[5]

The first comprehensive review of indications for TOE during cardiac surgery was published in 1996 by a task force of the American Society of Anesthesiologists and the Society of Cardiovascular Anesthesiologists.[5] This document has since been updated.[6] The indications are classified as Category I, IIa, IIb and III ; Category I indications include conditions for which there is evidence and/or general agreement that a given procedure or treatment is useful and effective (Table 7.1). Mitral valve repair, a surgical procedure performed with increasing frequency because of improved outcome compared to valve replacement, is an example of a Category I indication.[7,8] Echocardiographic evaluation involves describing the precise mechanism of regurgitation and designing repair prior to cardiopulmonary bypass. Following cardiopulmonary bypass the adequacy of the repair and any resulting complications including secondary stenosis and anterior leaflet ventricular outflow obstruction must be assessed (Fig. 7.1a, b, c). It can be a complex decision-making process which is performed by the cardiothoracic anaesthetist with increasing frequency. Close co-operation between surgeon and anaesthetist is required and interestingly it can significantly alter the nature of the traditional anaesthetist – surgeon relationship. Another Category I indication is placement of an intracardiac cannula. This is becoming increasingly common as more surgeons undertake minimally invasive cardiac surgery through a thoracotomy incision or use port access devices to avoid the use of an aortic cross-clamp. This indication also describes such procedures as accurate positioning of intra-aortic balloon counter-pulsation pumps and

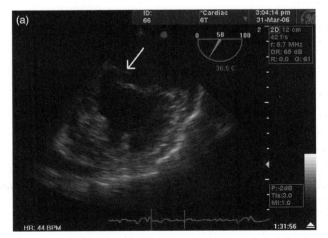

Fig. 7.1 Images captured during mitral valve repair: (a) the P3 scallop of the posterior mitral leaflet is seen to prolapse back into the left atrium during systole, producing a regurgitant orifice; (b) colour Doppler examination of the same patient demonstrates the resulting obliquely directed regurgitant jet (regurgitation produced by this mechanism is nearly always severe); (c) following repair the mitral annuloplasty ring can be seen; part of the prolapsing leaflet has also been resected, producing a competent mitral valve.

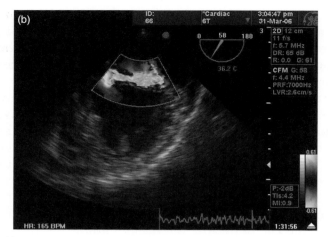

Fig. 7.1 (cont.)

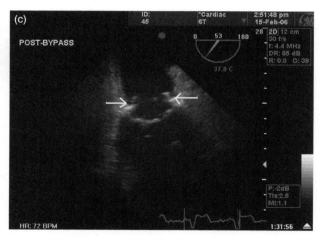

Fig. 7.1 (cont.)

coronary sinus catheters.[9,10] The first indication in Category I is evaluation of acute, persistent, and life-threatening hemodynamic disturbances. This encompasses a number of situations encountered in the cardiac operating theatre and critical care unit. Indeed, because of the powerful diagnostic ability of TOE (particularly in the ventilated patient), when immediately available, it is superior to institution of haemodynamic monitoring in indicating initial therapeutic interventions. Notably absent from the table of indications are valve replacement surgery and surgical coronary artery revascularisation. However, there is considerable evidence that intra-operative TOE can improve outcomes from these two types of cardiac surgery, particularly in circumstances where preoperative echocardiography is not readily available. There has been considerable debate as to whether intra-operative TOE is indicated as a routine monitor during coronary artery bypass surgery. The debate centres on the frequency with which this monitoring changes the nature of the surgical intervention, with quoted rates between 2.8% and 14.6%.[11,12,13,14,16] Haemodynamic interventions as a result of TOE findings may be considerably more frequent in coronary revascularisation therapy. In view of the low risk of morbidity and mortality of intra-operative TOE in comparison to invasive haemodynamic monitoring,[17,18] this author considers intra-operative TOE an effective routine monitoring tool for valve replacement and coronary artery surgery.

Intensive care

Clinical impact

Echocardiography is performed by cardiologists and echocardiology technicians in the vast majority of episodes in intensive care units (ICUs) in the UK. Recently there has been debate as to whether intensivists should take a more active role in developing and delivering this technology in the care of the critically ill[19,20,21] especially with the availability of more portable hand-held echocardiography platforms. The potential impact of echocardiography in the ICU is nicely demonstrated in a study where 36% of patients in a sample of 500 were diagnosed by transthoracic echocardiography (TTE) to have cardiac abnormalities, 77% of which were previously unsuspected.[22] Whereas TTE is normally the initial investigation, this may be limited by impaired views in the ventilated patient and there is good evidence that the diagnostic rate may be further improved by the use of the oesophageal window.[23] A comprehensive review of the impressive impact of TOE in a general surgical ICU demonstrated a diagnostic impact on 88% and a therapeutic impact on 68% of patients.[24] Using a structured educational programme, intensivists can be taught to perform a limited TOE examination, concentrating in particular on left ventricular loading and contractility. This is simple, safe and effective in the management of critically ill patients and provides alternative information to the pulmonary artery catheter (PAC).[25] Table 7.2 summarises the indications for echocardiography as a first-line diagnostic tool. Aortic dissection is a particular clinical situation where the whole patient management pathway has been changed by the advent of anaesthetic TOE practice. Computerised axial tomography (CAT) scanning and magnetic resonance imaging (MRI) were the standards for diagnosis of acute aortic dissection; the current generation of TOE scanners have a diagnostic capability which is at least as good as these techniques.[26,27,28,29] This enables rapid diagnosis in the emergency room or critical care unit as the

Table 7.2 Diagnostic indications for echocardiography in the intensive care unit.

The haemodynamically unstable patient
Hypoxaemia and respiratory failure
Pericardial disease
Massive pulmonary embolus
Investigation of unstable and complicated acute coronary syndromes
Evaluation of the multiple trauma patient
Evaluation of murmurs or suspected abnormal valve function
Investigation of sepsis of unknown origin and suspected endocarditis
Investigation of suspected aortic dissection
Source of stroke or distant embolisation
Diagnosis and drainage of pericardial and pleural effusions
Site of intravascular devices (intra-aortic balloon pump, pulmonary artery catheter)
Investigation of the patient with congenital heart disease or cardiopulmonary transplant

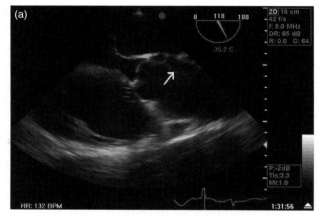

Fig. 7.2 (a) shows a long-axis view of the aortic root with dissected intimal flap (arrow); (b) shows an image of the same patient using colour flow Doppler: the false lumen is defined by absence of colour (arrow); (c) shows an image of the same patient in short axis with the intimal flap clearly visible; (d) shows the same view with colour doppler applied: the true and false lumens are clearly visible.

patient is prepared for theatre, and reduces the risks of a potentially hazardous trip to distant scanning areas. A further advantage is that presence of pericardial effusion and aortic valve incompetence can be confirmed as well as haemodynamic data and ventricular assessment (Fig. 7.2a, b, c, d). Echocardiography may also be useful in the investigation of the hypoxaemic patient in assessing right heart function, left ventricular (LV) loading conditions, intracardiac shunts and non-invasive measurement of pulmonary vascular pressures. With a short training period (using either a larger platform or a smaller hand-held unit) the immediate bedside diagnosis and drainage of pleural effusions is rapidly possible.

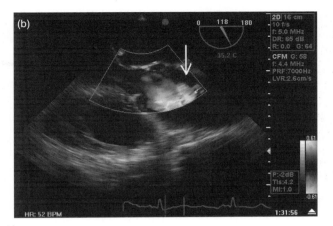

Fig. 7.2 (cont.)

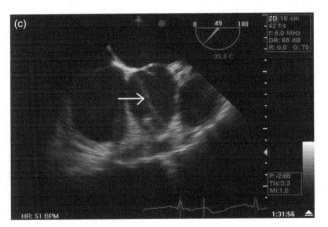

Fig. 7.2 (cont.)

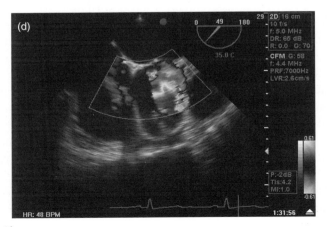

Fig. 7.2 (cont.)

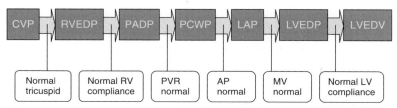

Fig. 7.3 Cardiac chamber measurements and assumptions: CVP = central venous pressure, RVEDP = right ventricular end-diastolic pressure, PADP = pulmonary artery diastolic pressure, PCWP = pulmonary capillary wedge pressure, LAP = left atrial pressure, LVEDP = left ventricular end-diastolic pressure, LVEDV = left ventricular end-diastolic volume, PVR = pulmonary vascular resistance, AP = airway pressure, MV = mitral valve.

Haemodynamic monitoring

Hypotension and consequent organ hypoperfusion is one of the common clinical problems in critically ill patients. Whilst there are numerous aetiologies and pathophysiological complexities that may give rise to this situation, most can be simplified into three categories: reduced intravascular volume, systemic vasodilatation and reduced cardiac contractility. The cornerstone of management of systemic hypoperfusion is intravascular pressure measurement, in particular measurement of central venous pressure and pulmonary arterial wedge pressure. There are, unfortunately, a significant number of assumptions that must be made for these measurements to accurately reflect LV end diastolic volume (LVEDV) (Fig. 7.3). There is a perception that pressure-based indices of ventricular loading compare unfavourably with echocardiographic-derived area/volume indices[30] and indeed the search goes on for a monitoring device with continuous capabilities.[31] Echocardiography can measure LVEDV or, more accurately, LV end-diastolic area (LVEDA) directly. Although there can be difficulties in the interpretation of this index, hypovolaemia in the patient without significant left ventricular impairment is relatively easy to assess. Echocardiography also enables direct visual assessment of left and right ventricular contractility, which cannot be obtained from any other current monitor, although oesophageal Doppler and pulse waveform analysis can provide an indirect assessment. Other cardiac indices that can be obtained include stroke volume and cardiac output, ejection fraction and fractional area change, LV diastolic function and tissue Doppler to assess the longitudinal contractile function of the ventricle. Furthermore pulmonary artery pressures can be derived and dynamic left ventricular outflow obstruction can be diagnosed (which may occur during inotrope therapy in critical care or non-cardiac surgery even in patients without hypertrophic obstructive cardiomyopathy).[32]

In summary, echocardiography provides an in-depth snapshot view of cardiac structures and haemodynamics in the critically ill patient, which leads to a significant therapeutic impact compared with currently used monitors together with a highly important diagnostic ability. There may be future improvements in its ability to predict pre-load responsiveness and its utility for continuous monitoring side by side with increasing educational opportunities for intensivists.

Non-cardiac surgery

Since the arrival of successful commercial TOE platforms in the cardiac theatres in the last two decades and their widespread uptake and impact, they are being wheeled along the corridor with increasing frequency to the non-cardiac theatres and the emergency department. Although there are still logistical limitations with availability of the required equipment and skills, the following is a summary of the indications and the possible uses of TOE in differing types of trauma and surgery.

Pre-assessment

Echocardiography has long been a valuable tool in the work-up of patients with cardiorespiratory dysfunction prior to non-cardiac surgery. This work is generally best done in consultation with cardiology colleagues. Whereas investigation of such conditions as aortic valvular stenosis is essential,[33] assessment of resting left ventricular function is a poor predictor of outcome.[34,35] Dobutamine-stress echocardiography may have more value as a predictor of a group of patients who have a high risk of perioperative ischaemic events.[36] With the recent interest in echocardiography by anaesthetists, screening echocardiography by anaesthetists in the pre-assessment clinic has proven valuable in reducing patient waits for surgery (personal communication). This may be facilitated by the recent availability of the hand-held echocardiography platforms.

Trauma

Blunt chest trauma is a particularly severe consequence of road traffic accidents and incurs a high mortality from haemmorhage and damage to cardiac structures and the great vessels. Owing to the unstable cardiovascular status of these patients they are hazardous to investigate in the scanner, and immediate diagnosis and intervention may improve outcomes. A prospective multicentre study in blunt chest trauma showed 56% of those evaluated by TOE had pathological findings, demonstrating the key role TOE may play in the management of these patients,[37] which has been recently confirmed by another study.[38] Transoesophageal echocardiography is particularly effective in the diagnosis of pericardial effusion and cardiac tamponade, myocardial contusion and aortic rupture and dissection.[39,40] For urgent investigation of penetrating cardiac trauma TTE is the preferable imaging modality as it demonstrates the anterior structures with greater clarity.

Vascular surgery

The main uses of TOE during major vascular surgery are pre-load and left ventricular function assessment together with myocardial ischaemia monitoring. Management changes of an order of 40% have been observed, in particular for volume therapy and inotrope and pressor agent use.[41] Although TOE detects myocardial ischaemia earlier and more accurately than electrocardiograph (ECG) (26% vs. 10%), studies have so far failed to demonstrate significant improvements in outcomes.[42,43,44,45] With the development of endovascular stents for aortic aneurysm repair, TOE has been valuable for demonstration of successful placement.[46]

Neurosurgery

Echocardiography is widely utilised in the pre-operative assessment of patients due to undergo craniotomy in the sitting position to detect the presence of patent foramen ovale and other right-to-left shunts. More recently TOE has been employed for the intra-operative detection and treatment of venous air embolism in the sitting position. The incidence of this complication is up to 45% in patients undergoing this procedure.[47] The use of TOE allows detection of air bubbles down to 1 mm in diameter; furthermore it assists in the placement of an air aspiration catheter and allows immediate monitoring of ventricular function.[48]

Orthopaedic surgery

Although TOE is not a routine monitor in major joint replacement surgery, its ability to demonstrate embolic events (fat, thrombus and air) during the insertion of cemented hip prosthesis and subsequent joint reduction has been clearly demonstrated.[49,50] This can result in significant cardio-respiratory morbidity and together with the cardiovascular co-morbidities in the ageing surgical population a role for intra-operative TOE may be clarified in the future.

Liver transplantation

The value of TOE during orthotopic liver transplantation has been demonstrated in the management of pre-load, ventricular dysfunction and embolic events that occur with the postreperfusion syndrome.[51,52,53,54,55]

Training and accreditation in TOE

Training

The factors which have limited the more widespread uptake of TOE as a monitor and diagnostic tool, particularly in the general operating theatre and the intensive care unit, are the relative expense and the perceived complexity of the technology, as well as the lack of comprehensive training programmes. Whereas a cardiologist in training will have early and continued exposure to TTE throughout the term of his training, trainee anaesthetists will have relatively little exposure to TOE, unless they elect to do a cardiac anaesthesia fellowship. As a consultant anaesthetist it can be very difficult to gain sufficient exposure and training alongside the normal working responsibilities. The learning curve for perioperative TOE is longer than for comparable monitors such as oesophageal Doppler or the pulmonary artery catheter. This is in part because mastery of the different ultrasound modes (M-mode, 2-D scanning, colour flow Doppler and spectral Doppler) requires considerable practice, and in part because of the time taken to gain exposure to the wide variety of pathological lesions. The basic level of training in the USA, as specified by the SCA/ASE guidelines (Society of Cardiovascular Anesthesiologists/ American Society of Echocardiography), requires 150 completed examinations, and advanced training requires more than 300 examinations.[1] Defined sets of cognitive and technical skills required for proficiency have been published.[56] Despite the commitment required to achieve TOE competence, a survey of Canadian anaesthesiologists in training indicate that up to 40% would rather learn TOE than pursue an academic programme during residency.[57] A number of short courses, at a basic skills level, with an emphasis on practical 'hands-on' experience have existed for a few years in the UK. These have proved very popular with a wide variety of sub-specialists, from cardiothoracic anaesthetists to intensivists and liver transplant anaesthetists. Ultimately the factors determining long-term likelihood of achieving competence for these interested parties will be availability of equipment and technical and knowledge back-up from cardiologists and cardiothoracic anaesthetists and other interested practitioners. There is a need for more research into educational methods for acquiring complex skills such as TOE. There are as yet no simulator methods, as in other fields of anaesthesia, developed for TOE training.

Accreditation

North America
Just prior to its publication of practice guidelines for intra-operative TOE,[5] the Society of Cardiovascular Anesthesiologists (the Cardiothoracic Anesthesiologists Society in the United States of America) created a task force to implement and design an assessment test for perioperative trans-oesophageal echocardiography (PTE). The examination was piloted in 1997 and the first official examination was offered in 1998. The PTE examination subcommittee, together with a committee from the ASE,

was co-opted as part of the National Board of Echocardiography (NBE) – which administers other examinations in echocardiographic competency. This then became the first examination process in the world using which anaesthetist echocardiographers could compare their knowledge against an established standard. In addition to their North American counterparts, cardiothoracic anaesthetists, particularly from the United Kingdom, Australia and mainland Europe, travelled to gain this PTE diploma. Pass rates for the first four years of between 72–84% were established. Over the subsequent years the NBE has expanded the process to become a board-certified competency process – as well as passing the examination, candidates must also submit a logbook with 150 cases. From 2008 the NBE has decreed that certification of competency can only be attained as part of a recognised cardiothoracic anaesthesia fellowship programme.[58,59,60]

United Kingdom

Anaesthetist-delivered intra-operative TOE in the UK evolved from certain highly specialised cardiothoracic surgical centres such as Harefield Hospital. A small number of specialist anaesthetists trained in the USA and imparted their knowledge and experience to colleagues and trainees. From a small number of practical intra-operative courses other cardiothoracic centres in the UK established intra-operative TOE services provided by anaesthetists. As anaesthetic interest increased and surgical requests likewise surged, a demand for a home-grown process of accreditation arose. The Association of Cardiothoracic Anaesthetists (ACTA) established a TOE subcommittee in 1998 to oversee the quality of intra-operative TOE education. From this a Task Force on Certification for Perioperative TOE published a syllabus for basic TOE knowledge. Prior to these events, the cardiologists' sub-specialist professional body, the British Society of Echocardiography (BSE), had a well-established accreditation in adult TTE. Keen to consolidate the role of the anaesthetist echocardiographer, ACTA embarked on a co-operative venture with the BSE to develop a formal TOE accreditation. Developing on this experience and incorporating the lessons of the North American process, the first TOE examination resulting from this joint consultation was held in 2003. After a considerable period of discussion, the ACTA/BSE accreditation in TOE now requires the written examination together with a record of 125 reported cases gathered within a period of two years, as well as a number of video case reports. This competency is open to cardiologists, anaesthetists, sonographers, intensivists, and in fact anyone whose professional practice includes TOE. The examination is now held bi-annually and the accreditation process is now established. Future projects include departmental accreditation for TOE in line with accreditation for departmental TTE accreditation.[61,62,63]

Europe and Australasia

In Europe there has been a similar co-operation between the European Association of Cardiothoracic Anaesthetists (EACTA) and the European Society of Echocardiography (ESE). This has lead to an accreditation process very similar to that developed in the UK; in fact some of the team that developed the UK accreditation have also been instrumental in the European process. The language of the examination is currently English, although there are plans to establish other language versions depending on uptake. There is no accreditation per se in Australia and New Zealand. Australian anaesthetists or intensivist echocardiographers have previously travelled to the USA to sit the SCA/ASE examination. More recently a postgraduate diploma in perioperative and critical care echocardiography has been offered from Melbourne University, which is predominantly a correspondence course. Both these qualifications are recognised by the Australian and New Zealand College of Anaesthetists along with recommended training periods and case numbers to demonstrate competence.

Technology

A brief history

Medical ultrasound had its origins in the development of sonar technology to detect submarines. Clinical echocardiography as we know it was developed in Sweden in the 1950s. The earliest scans were M-mode and subsequently 2-dimensional and Doppler applications were developed for transthoracic echocardiography (TTE). Transoesophageal echocardiography (TOE) developed in the 1970s by mounting a transducer on an endoscope; TOE probes have the same scanning and Doppler capabilities as TTE probes. Intravascular ultrasound transducers mounted on cardiac catheters have been around since the 1970s. More recently there has been the development of real time three-dimensional and hand-held echocardiography.

Recent developments in imaging technology

Echocardiography probes

The first generation of TOE probes were monoplane probes which, like their TTE equivalents, possessed only one fixed scanning plane. These were followed by the bi-plane probe, which was rapidly succeeded by the omniplane probe, which has now become the clinical standard TOE probe. The omniplane probe contains a motor in the tip which rotates the transducer through 180 degrees allowing a detailed sweep of any structures of interest. There is also a smaller paediatric TOE probe available, which allows the intubation of children for scanning purposes. Another development in intra-operative scanning is the use of epi-aortic probes which can assist in the identification of atheromatous plaques in the ascending aorta and has been shown to reduce the incidence of cerebrovascular injury following cardiac surgery.[64] This technique is ready for re-evaluation with the establishment of off-pump coronary artery surgery and new devices for coronary anastamosis which avoid the need for an aortic cross-clamp. At the same time TTE scanning has been improved by the development of harmonic imaging. Intravascular probes are intracardiac catheter-size probes which can be inserted through the femoral or other large vein allowing visualisation of intracardiac structures; this has proved particularly useful for scanning during closure of atrial septal defects and for exploration of the atria during catheter ablation of atrial arrhythmias.[65,66]

Tissue doppler

For tissue Doppler studies, the myocardium can be imaged by using pulsed-Doppler echocardiography and filtering high velocities to obtain a signal. This can be measured near the mitral annulus and is sometimes also known as the mitral annulus velocity. The tissue Doppler allows the left ventricular relaxation rate to be measured independently of pre-load. The typical pattern in diastole is similar to the mitral flow pattern with an early (E_m) wave and atrial (A_m) wave. Because of its pre-load independence, it can be used to obtain filling pressure from the left ventricular filling pattern and has been validated against invasive measurements of left atrial pressure measurement.[67,68,69]

Contrast echocardiography

Contrast echocardiography can significantly improve definition of the endo-cardial border and thus significantly improve assessment of left ventricular wall contractility, which is particularly valuable in the 10–20% of studies in which this may be technically difficult. The microbubble technology used for intravascular echocardiography contrast has also improved the ability of stress echocardiography to detect myocardial ischaemia (Fig. 7.4).[70,71,72]

Three-dimensional echocardiography

Three-dimensional (3-D) echocardiography is one of the most exciting recent developments in echocardiography. Originally developed in the 1980s, this technology has made the leap into clinical reality in the last five years. Three-dimensional imaging was first developed as an offline reconstruction of 2-D imaging; now with the improvement in matrix array transducers, real-time 3-D imaging has arrived. This has been well validated against cardiac magnetic resonance imaging (another rapidly developing field) for the accurate assessment of left ventricular morphology

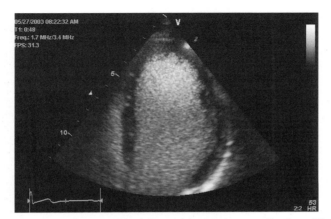

Fig. 7.4 Contrast echocardiogram of the left ventricle showing opacification of the ventricular cavity and imaging enhancement of the ventricular walls.

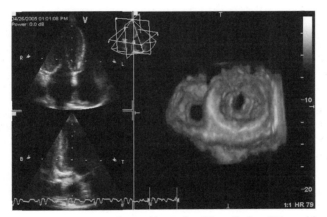

Fig. 7.5 Three-dimensional echocardiographic study of the mitral and tricuspid valves.

and function.[73,74,75] Real-time 3-D imaging offers promising advances in the understanding of functional mitral valve regurgitation and ventricular geometry, with the possibility of new treatments.[76] Real-time 3-D TOE has not yet made the same advances as TTE; however, the use of 3-D reconstructions of 2-D TOE imaging suggests surgical advances may be possible with advances in this technology (Fig. 7.5).[77]

Hand-held echocardiography

Lightweight portable echocardiography units have been in existence since the 1970s but have suffered in terms of image quality and digital storage in comparison to the larger laboratory-based machines. There has been an upsurge in interest in these machines and several are now aimed at the intensive care market. These machines range in price and sophistication

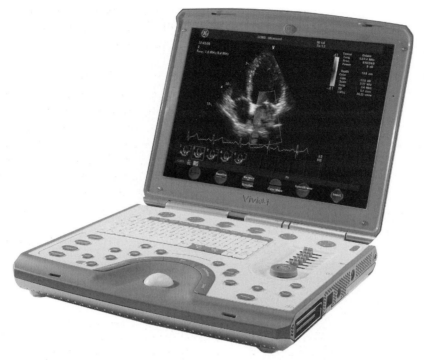

Fig. 7.6 The vivid-*i*, one of the new laptop-based portable echocardiographic systems. The performance and applications of these scanners can rival those of the large laboratory-based systems despite its compact size.

from the simple machines which can be used for screening echocardiography to the fully functional laptop-based replacement for top-end scanners (Fig. 7.6). One of the companies working together with a manufacturer of anaesthetic machines has developed a mobile side arm for portable echo machines to be locked on to for use in the theatre.

Conclusion

Echocardiography technology has had a remarkable and sustained development in clinical applications and technological progress, particularly in recent years. Advances in computer technology enable continued miniaturisation and enhanced image quality and this process can only accelerate in the future. All units now available have digital images which are increasingly stored in huge online data storage banks; wireless connectivity should hopefully solve the data storage problems with portable echocardiography. The most exciting development in imaging is 3-D echocardiography. Whilst this is in the early stages of its clinical life, technological advances will mean that new insights into ventricular geometry and valve function can lead to new treatments and surgical interventions. When high quality 3-D TOE is developed this will enable detailed intra-operative assessment, enabling development of new valve-repair techniques.

For the anaesthetists and intensivists of the future, echocardiography will be increasingly important technology. Training courses are now available and a new generation of 'perioperative physician' trainees who are competent in its use will arise. The inevitable increase in the use of anaesthetic preoperative assessment clinics will provide anaesthetists with the opportunity to develop screening echocardiography skills. This 'one-stop shop' will reduce delays in surgical waiting time and at the same time allow anaesthetists greater ownership of the preoperative patient journey. Similarly in the intra-operative and ICU environments there will be less demand on cardiology colleagues and improved clinical decision-making as echocardiography becomes an important and readily available monitor for patients with cardiovascular co-morbidities.

References

1. Shanewise JS, Cheung AT, Aronson S, *et al*. ASE/SCA Guidelines for Performing a Comprehensive Intraoperative Multiplane Transesophageal Echocardiography Examination: Recommendations of the American Society of Echocardiography Council for Intraoperative Echocardiography and the Society of Cardiovascular Anesthesiologists Task Force for Certification in Perioperative Transesophageal Echocardiography. *Anesth Analg* 1999; **89**: 870–84.
2. Flachskampf FA, Decoodt P, Fraser AG, *et al*. Guidelines from the Working Group: Recommendations for Performing Transoesophageal Echocardiography. *Eur J Echocardiogr* 2001; **2**: 8–21.
3. Morewood GH, Gallagher ME, Gaughan JP, Conlay LA. Current practice patterns for adult perioperative transoesophageal echocardiography in the United States. *Anaesthesiology* 2001; **95**: 1507–12.
4. Lambert AS, Mazer CD, Duke PC. Survey of the members of the cardiovascular section of the Canadian Anesthesiologists' Society on the use of perioperative transesophageal echocardiography – a brief report. *Can J Anesth* 2002; **49**: 294–6.
5. Thys DM, Abel M, Bollen BA, *et al*. Practice guidelines for perioperative transesophageal echocardiography: a report by the American Society of Anesthesiologists and the Society of Cardiovascular Anesthesiologists Task Force on Transesophageal Echocardiography. *Anesthesiology* 1996; **84**: 986–1006.
6. Cheitlin MD, Armstrong WF, Aurigemma GP, *et al*. ACC/AHA/ASE 2003 Guideline Update for the Clinical Application of Echocardiography: Summary Article: A Report of the American College of Cardiology/American Heart Association Task Force on Practice Guidelines (ACC/AHA/ASE Committee to Update the 1997 Guidelines for the Clinical Application of Echocardiography). *Circulation* 2003; **108**: 1146–62.
7. Savage EB, Ferguson TB Jr, DiSesa VJ. Use of mitral valve repair: analysis of contemporary United States experience reported to the Society of

Thoracic Surgeons National Cardiac Database. *Ann Thorac Surg* 2003; **75**: 820–5.

8. Braunberger E, Deloche A, Berrebi A, *et al*. Very long-term results (more than 20 years) of valve repair with Carpentier's techniques in nonrheumatic mitral valve insufficiency. *Circulation* 2001; **104**(Suppl 1): I-8–I-11.

9. Shih CT, Yang MW, Lai ST, Lin CY. Early detection of the tip position and complication of the intra-aortic balloon pump catheter by perioperative transesophageal echocardiography. *Chin Med J* 1994; **53**: 131–4.

10. Demirsoy E, Ozbek U, Bayindir O, Sonmez B. Clinical experience with coronary sinus catheterization in minimally invasive aortic valve surgery under transeso-phageal echocardiography guidance. *Int J Cardiovasc Imaging* 2002; **18**: 453–5.

11. Savage R, Lytle B, Aronson S, *et al*. Intraoperative echocardiography is indi-cated in high-risk coronary artery bypass grafting. *Ann Thorac Surg* 1997; **64**: 368–74.

12. Mishra M, Chauhan R, Sharma K, *et al*. Real-time intraoperative echocardiography – how useful? Experience of 5,016 cases. *J Cardiothorac Vasc Anesth* 1998; **112**: 625–32.

13. Click R, Abel M, Schaff H. Intraoperative transesophageal echocardiography: 5-year prospective review of impact on surgical management. *Mayo Clin Proc* 2000; **75**: 241–47.

14. Schmidlin D, Bettex D, Bernard E, *et al*. Transoesophageal echocardiography in cardiac and vascular surgery: implications and observer variability. *Br J Anaesth* 2001; **86**: 497–501.

15. Couture P, Denault A, McKenty S, *et al*. Impact of routine use of intraoperative transesophageal echocardiography during cardiac surgery. *Can J Anesth* 2000; **47**: 20–6.

16. Lovelock N, Forrest P, Hu J, Fletcher SN. The impact of intraoperative trans-oesophageal echocardiography on an unselected cardiac surgical population: a review of 2,343 cases. *Anaesth Intens Care* 2002; **30**: 734–41.

17. Harvey S, Harrison DA, Singer M, *et al*. Assessment of the clinical effectiveness of pulmonary artery catheters in management of patients in intensive care (PAC-Man): a randomised controlled trial. *Lancet* 2005; **366**: 472–7.

18. Kallmeyer I, Collard C, Fox J, *et al*. The safety of intraoperative transesopha-geal echocardiography: a case series of 7200 cardiac surgical patients. *Anesth Analg* 2001; **92**: 1126–30.

19. Kitching A, Fielden J. Bringing the mountain to Mohamed: Echocardiography in the ICU. *Care Critically Ill* 2002; **18**: 72–3.

20. Ketzler JT, McSweeney ME, Coursin DB. ICU echocardiography: should we use it in a heartbeat? *Chest* 2002; **122**: 1121–3.

21. Colreavy FB, Donovan K, Lee K Y, Weekes J. Transesophageal echocardio-graphy in critically ill patients. *Crit Care Med* 2002; **30**: 989–96.

22. Bossone E, Giovine B, Watts S, *et al*. Range and prevalence of cardiac abnormalities in patients hospitalized in a medical ICU. *Chest* 2002; **122**: 1370–6.

23. Vignon P, Mentec H, Terre S, *et al*. Diagnostic accuracy and therapeutic impact of transthoracic and transoesophageal echocardiography in mechanically ventilated patients in the ICU. *Chest* 1994; **106**: 1829–34.

24. Huttemann E, Schelenz C, Kara F, Chatzinikolaou K, Reinhart K. The use and safety of transoesophageal echocardiography in the general ICU – a minireview. *Acta Anaesthesiol Scand* 2004; **48**: 827–36.

25. Benjamin E, Griffin K, Leibowitz AB, *et al*. Goal-directed transesophageal echocardiography performed by intensivists to assess left ventricular function: comparison with pulmonary artery catheterization. *J Cardiothorac Vasc Anesth* 1998; **12**: 10–15.

26. Erbel R, Daniel W, Visser C, *et al*. Echocardiography in diagnosis of aortic dissection. *Lancet* 1989; **1**: 457–69.

27. Nienaber CA, Spielmann RP, von Kodolitsch Y, *et al*. Diagnosis of thoracic aortic dissection: magnetic resonance imaging versus transesophageal echocardiography. *Circulation*; **85**: 434–47.

28. Simon P, Owen AN, Havel M, *et al*. Transesophageal echocardiography in the emergency surgical management of patients with aortic dissection. *J Thorac Cardiovasc Surg* 1992; **103**: 1113–18.

29. Laissy JP, Blanc F, Soyer P, *et al*. Thoracic aortic dissection: diagnosis with transesophageal echocardiography versus MR imaging. *Radiology* 1995; **194**: 331–6.

30. Kumar A, Anel R, Bunnell E, *et al*. Pulmonary artery occlusion pressure and central venous pressure fail to predict ventricular filling volume, cardiac performance, or the response to volume infusion in normal subjects. *Crit Care Med* 2004; **32**: 691–9.

31. Hofer CK, Ganter MT, Matter-Ensner, *et al*. Volumetric assessment of left heart pre-load by thermodilution: comparing the PiCCO-VoLEF®system with transoesophageal echocardiography. *Anaesthesia* 2006; **61**: 316–21.

32. Luckner G, Margreiter J, Jochberger S, *et al*. Systolic anterior motion of the mitral valve with left ventricular outflow tract obstruction: three cases of acute perioperative hypotension in noncardiac surgery. *Anesth Analg* 2005; **100**: 1594–8.

33. Christ M, Sharkova Y, Geldner G, Maisch B. Preoperative and perioperative care for patients with suspected or established aortic stenosis facing noncardiac surgery. *Chest* 2005; **128**: 2944–53.

34. Halm EA, Browner WS, Tubau JF, *et al*. Echocardiography for assessing cardiac risk in patients having noncardiac surgery. *Ann Intern Med* 1996; **125**: 433–41.

35. Rhode LE, Polanczyk CA, Goldman L, *et al*. Usefulness of transthoracic echocardiography as a tool for risk stratification of patients undergoing major noncardiac surgery. *Am J Cardiol* 2001; **87**: 505–9.

36. Boersma E, Poldermans D, Bax JJ, *et al*. Predictors of cardiac events after major vascular surgery. Role of clinical characteristics, dobutamine echocardiography and ß-blocker therapy. *JAMA* 2001; **285**: 1865–73.

37. Garcia-Fernandez MA, Lopez-Perez JM, Perez-Castellano, *et al*. Role of transesophageal echocardiography in the assessment of patients with blunt chest trauma: correlation of echocardiographic findings with the electrocardiogram and creatine kinase monoclonal antibody measurements. *Am Heart J* 1998; **135**: 476–81.

38. Burns JM, Sing RF, Mostafa G, *et al*. The role of transesophageal echocardiography in optimizing resuscitation in acutely injured patients. *J Trauma* 2005; **59**: 36–42.

39. Weiss RL, Brier JA, O'Connor W, *et al*. The usefulness of transesophageal echocardiography in diagnosing cardiac contusions. *Chest* 1996; **109**: 73–7.

40. Saletta S, Lederman E, Fein S, *et al*. Transoesophageal echocardiography for the initial evaluation of the widened mediastinum in trauma patients. *J Trauma* 1995; **39**: 137–42.

41. Denault NY, Couture P, McKenty S, *et al*. Perioperative use of transoesophageal echocardiography by anesthesiologists: impact in non-cardiac surgery and in the intensive care unit. *Can J Anesth* 2002; **49**: 287–93.

42. Krupski WC, Layug EL, Reilly LM, *et al*. Comparison of cardiac morbidity between aortic and infrainguinal operations. Study of perioperative ischaemia (SPI) research group. *J Vasc Surg* 1992; **15**: 354–63.

43. Krupski WC, Layug EL, Reilly LM, *et al*. Comparison of cardiac morbidity rates between aortic and infrainguinal operations: two-year follow up. Study of perioperative ischaemia (SPI) research group. *J Vasc Surg* 1993; **18**: 605–19.

44. London MJ, Tubau JF, Wong MG, *et al*. The natural history of segmental wall motion abnormalities in patients undergoing non-cardiac surgery. *Anesthesiology* 1990; **73**: 644–55.

45. Eisenberg MJ, London MJ, Leung JM, *et al*. Monitoring for myocardial ischaemia during non-cardiac surgery. A technology assessment of transesophageal echocardiography and 12 lead electrocardiography. *JAMA* 1992; **268**: 210–16.

46. Moskowitz DM, Kahn RA, Konstadt SN, *et al*. Intraoperative transesophageal echocardiography as an adjuvant to fluoroscopy during endovascular thoracic aortic repair. *Eur J Vasc Endovasc Surg* 1999; **17**: 22–7.

47. Gottlieb JD, Ericsson JA, Sweet RB. Venous air embolism: a review. *Anesth Analg* 1965; **44**: 773–9.

48. Reeves ST, Bevis LA, Bailey BN. Positioning a right atrial air aspiration catheter using transesophageal echocardiography. *J Neurosurg Anesthesiol* 1996; **8**: 123–5.

49. Koessler MJ, Fabiani R, Hamer H, *et al*. The clinical relevance of embolic events detected by transesophageal echocardiography during cemented total hip arthroplasty: a randomized clinical trial. *Anesth Analg* 2001; **92**: 49–55.

50. Johnson C, Lewis KD, Steen SN, *et al*. Transesophageal echocardiography in the anesthetic management of total hip arthroplasty. *Acta Anesthesiol Sin* 2001; **39**: 135–8.

51. Hofer CK, Zollinger A, Rak M, *et al*. Therapeutic impact of intraoperative transoesophageal echocardiography during noncardiac surgery. *Anaesthesia* 2004; **59**: 3–9.

52. Krenn CG, Hoda R, Nikolic A, *et al*. Assessment of ventricular contractile function during orthotopic liver transplantation. *Transpl Int* 2004; **17**: 101–4.

53. Planinsic RM, Nicolau-Raducu R, Caldwell JC, Aggarwal S, Hilmi I. Transesophageal echocardiography-guided placement of internal jugular percutaneous venovenous bypass cannula in orthotopic liver transplantation. *Anesth Analg* 2003; **97**: 648–9.

54. Schumann R. Intraoperative resource utilization in anesthesia for liver transplantation in the United States: a survey. *Anesth Analg* 2003; **97**: 21–8.

55. Feierman D. Case presentation: transesophageal echocardiography during orthotopic liver transplantation – not only a different diagnosis, but different management. *Liver Transpl Surg* 1999; **5**: 340–1.

56. Thys D. Clinical competence in echocardiography. *Anesth Analg* 2003; **97**: 313–22.

57. Silcox LC, Ashbury TL, Van Den Kerkhof EG, Milne B. Residents' and program directors' attitudes toward research during anesthesiology training: a Canadian perspective. *Anesth Analg* 2006; **102**: 859–64.

58. Weyman AE, Butler A, Subhiyah R, *et al*. Concept, development, administration and analysis of a certifying examination in echocardiography for physicians. *J Am Soc Echocardiogr* 2001; **14**: 158–68.

59. Cahalan MK, Abel M, Goldman M, *et al*. American Society of Echocardiography and Society of Cardiovascular Anaesthetists Task Force Guidelines for training in perioperative echocardiography. *Anesth Analg* 2002; **94**: 1384–8.

60. Aronson S, Butler A, Subhiyah R, *et al*. Development and analysis of a new certifying examination in perioperative transoesophageal echocardiography. *Anesth Analg* 2002; **95**: 1476–82.

61. Swanevelder J, Chin D, Kneeshaw J, *et al*. Accreditation in transoesophageal echocardiography: a statement from the Association of Cardiothoracic Anaesthetists and the British Society of Echocardiography Joint TOE Accreditation Committee. *Br J Anaesth* 2003; **91**: 469–72.

62. Wright SJ, Barnard MJ, Smith A, *et al*. Accreditation in transoesophageal echocardiography. *Br J Anaesth* 2004; **92**: 446–8.

63. Riedel B, Shaw A, Thakar D. Accreditation in transoesophageal echocardiography. *Br J Anaesth* 2004; **93**: 2.

64. Davila-Roman VG, Barzilai B, Wareing TH, *et al*. Intraoperative ultrasonographic evaluation of the ascending aorta in 100 consecutive patients undergoing cardiac surgery. *Circulation* 1991; **84**: 47–53.

65. Gianluca R. Expanding the use of intracardiac echocardiography in congenital heart disease catheter-based interventions. *J Am Soc Echocardiogr* 2005; **18**: 1230.

66. Rotter M, Sanders P, Jais P, *et al*. Prospective validation of phased array intracardiac echocardiography for the assessment of atrial mechanical function during catheter ablation of atrial fibrillation. *Heart* 2006; **92**: 407–9.

67. Nagueh SF, Mikati I, Kopelen HA, *et al*. Doppler estimation of left ventricular filling pressure in sinus tachycardia: a new application of tissue doppler imaging. *Circulation* 1998; **98**: 1644–50.

68. Nagueh SF, Middleton KJ, Kopelen HA, *et al*. Doppler tissue imaging: a non invasive technique for evaluation of left ventricular relaxation and estimation of filling pressures. *J Am Coll Cardiol* 1997; **30**: 1527–33.

69. Sundereswaran L, Nagueh SF, Vardan S, *et al*. Estimation of left and right ventricular filling pressures after heart transplantation by tissue Doppler imaging. *Am J Cardiol* 1998; **82**: 352–7.

70. Cohen JL, Cheirif J, Segar DS, *et al*. Improved left ventricular endocardial border delineation and opacification with OPTISON (FS069), a new echocardiographic contrast agent. Results of a phase III multicentre trial. *J Am Coll Cardiol* 1998; **32**: 746–52.

71. Cheng S-C, Dy TC, Feinstein SB. Contrast echocardiography: review and future directions. *Am J Cardiol* 1998; **81**(12A):41–8G.

72. Cwajg J, Xie F, O'Leary E, *et al*. Detection of angiographically significant coronary artery disease with accelerated intermittent imaging after intravenous administration of ultrasound contrast material. *Am Heart J* 2000; **139**: 675–83.

73. Kuhl HP, Schreckenberg M, Rulands D, *et al*. High-resolution transthoracic real-time three-dimensional echocardiography: quantification of cardiac volumes and function using semi-automatic border detection and comparison with cardiac magnetic resonance imaging. *J Am Coll Cardiol* 2004; **43**: 23–9.

74. Zhuang L, Wang XF, Xie MX, *et al.* Experimental study of quantitative assessment of left ventricular mass with contrast enhanced real-time three-dimensional echocardiography. *J Am Coll Cardiol* 2004; **43**: 23–9.
75. Jenkins C, Bricknell K, Hanekom L, Marwick TH. Reproducibility and accuracy of echocardiographic measurements of left ventricular parameters using real-time three-dimensional echocardiography. *J Am Coll Cardiol*; **44**: 878–86.
76. Kwan J, Shiota T, Agler DA, *et al.* Geometric differences of the mitral apparatus between ischaemic and dilated cardiomyopathy with significant mitral regurgitation: real-time three-dimensional echocardiography study. *Circulation* 2003; **107**: 1135–40.
77. Macnab A, Jenkins NP, Bridgewater BJ, *et al.* Three-dimensional echocardiography is superior to multiplanetransoesophageal echo in the assessment of regurgitant mitral valve morphology. *Eur J Echocardiogr* 2004; **5**: 212–22.

CHAPTER 8

Scott Mercer and Andrew Rhodes

Levosimendan

Calcium sensitisers are a new class of positive inotropic drugs that are potentially useful in the treatment of acute decompensated heart failure. They have a unique mechanism of action that differs from other available intravenous agents such as dobutamine, a β-agonist, and milrinone, a phosphodiesterase inhibitor. Unlike dobutamine and milrinone, calcium sensitisers increase myocardial contractility without increasing cytosolic calcium release, reducing myocardial energy demand and the incidence of serious arrhythmias. Clinical trials have focused on demonstrating improved survival with levosimendan when compared to placebo and dobutamine. Levosimendan is the first intravenous calcium sensitiser to be approved in Europe for the treatment of acute decompensated heart failure.

Pharmacology

Chemical structure

Levosimendan is a pyridazinone-dinitrile derivative with the chemical name ((R) − (4-(1,4,5,6-tetrahydro-4-methyl-6-oxo-3-pyridazinyl)-phenyl)-hydrazono)propanedinitrile. Levosimendan is the levo-isomer of the racemic compound simendan. It is moderately lipophilic with a small molecular weight (280.29) and is a weak acid (pKa 6.26).

Pharmacological action

β-adrenergic agonists and phosphodiesterase inhibitors produce positive inotropic effects by increasing intracellular concentrations of free calcium.

Recent Advances in Anaesthesia and Intensive Care 24, ed. J. N. Cashman and R. M. Grounds.
Published by Cambridge University Press. © Cambridge University Press 2007.

This energy-dependent process involves increasing the intracellular concentration of cyclic adenosine monophosphate (cAMP).[1] Levosimendan has a dual mechanism of action, acting as a positive inotrope and a vasodilator. The positive inotropic effect of levosimendan is achieved by calcium sensitisation rather than increasing intracellular free calcium concentration, therefore avoiding the energy-dependent process. Levosimendan binds to cardiac troponin C and stabilises the conformational changes of troponin C, facilitating actin-myosin cross-bridge formation.[2,3,4] This binding occurs in a calcium concentration-dependent manner. At higher concentrations, levosimendan selectively inhibits phosphodiesterase-3, further augmenting these inotropic effects.[5,6,7]

An early concern regarding the use of calcium sensitisers was that they would impair ventricular relaxation by delaying the dissociation of calcium from the complex. Binding occurs in a concentration-dependent manner so that during systole, calcium concentrations are high and as a result levosimendan is more active.[4] Conversely during diastole, calcium concentrations are lower and levosimendan is inactive. Therefore, levosimendan does not impair relaxation.[5,8] Intracellular release of calcium is responsible for the pro-arrhythmogenic effects of current inotropes. Levosimendan does not appear to have the same arrhythmogenic potential because it acts by enhancing calcium sensitivity. The vasodilatory effects of levosimendan are attributed to the opening of K_{ATP} channels.[9] Levosimendan improves left ventricular systolic function and myocardial efficiency by increasing coronary blood flow and coronary vasodilation.[10]

Pharmacokinetics

The pharmacokinetics of levosimendan follows a two-compartment model with first-order elimination.[11] It undergoes rapid distribution and has a terminal elimination half-life of about 1 hour. The volume of distribution of levosimendan is approximately $0.2\,L.kg^{-1}$. Levosimendan is 97–98% bound to plasma proteins, primarily to albumin. The protein binding of the biologically active metabolite of levosimendan (OR-1896) is 40%.

Levosimendan is completely metabolised by two pathways. The main route of metabolism involves glutathione conjugation of levosimendan to biologically inactive cyclic or N-acetylated cysteine or cysteineglycine derivatives. The other minor route of metabolism actually results in the formation of the active metabolite. Levosimendan is reduced to an inactive metabolite (OR-1855) in the lower gastrointestinal tract. This is reabsorbed and acetylated to the biologically active metabolite (OR-1896). The pharmacological profile of OR-1896 resembles that of its parent compound levosimendan. Both OR-1855 and OR-1896 are formed slowly and have long elimination half-lives. Peak plasma concentrations are reached about two days after termination of the levosimendan infusion. It is believed that OR-1896 $(t_{0.5} = 81 \pm 37\,h)^{12}$ is responsible for the prolonged haemodynamic effects after elimination of the parent drug levosimendan.[13]

The clearance of levosimendan and OR-1896 is unaffected by renal impairment in patients with heart failure.[14,15] The percentage of the dose excreted in urine is 0.022% for levosimendan and less than 2% for the metabolites.[15] There is no information on the effects of hepatic impairment on clearance of levosimendan.

Clinical evidence

There have been a number of large, multicentred studies comparing levosimendan with dobutamine and with placebo in the treatment of acute decompensated heart failure. The results of all of the trials published so far are presented below and summarised in Table 8.1.

The LIDO study

The LIDO (Levosimendan Infusion versus DObutamine) study demonstrated superior outcomes for improving cardiac output, pulmonary catheter wedge pressure (PCWP) and short- and long-term survival with levosimendan when compared to dobutamine.[16] During the first 24 hours, there was similar improvement in cardiac output, but a rapid and more sustained decrease in PCWP in the levosimendan group. At 24 hours, the haemodynamic values were significantly improved with levosimendan versus dobutamine. Patients included in the study had moderate to severe heart failure. Half of the patients had ischaemic cardiomyopathy and some were awaiting heart transplantation (levosimendan 18%, dobutamine 15%). The study demonstrated sustained improvement in survival with levosimendan at 31 days and six months. The protocol was amended to evaluate all-cause mortality at 180 days. The explicit cause of death was not specified (e.g. heart failure, myocardial infarction, sudden death).

Patient self-assessment of dyspnoea and fatigue was done using a four-point scale (much better, slightly better, no change or worse). Ratings of fatigue and dyspnoea were similar between the two groups, with 68% of levosimendan and 59% of dobutamine patients reporting improved symptoms $(p = 0.865)$. Despite statistical difference in haemodynamic end points, the two drugs have similar impact on symptom improvement. The investigators performed a sub-group analysis in one-third of the

Table 8.1 Summary of clinical trials.

Study	Design	Treatment	Patient group	End points	Results
LIDO[16] (2002) ($n = 203$)	Randomised, placebo-controlled	Levosimendan: 24 mcg.kg^{-1} + 0.1 mcg.kg^{-1}.min^{-1} (dose doubled if response not seen at h) Dobutamine: 5 mcg.kg^{-1}.min^{-1}	Low-output heart failure requiring haemodynamic monitoring and an iv inotrope, EF ≤ 30%, PCWP ≥ 15 mmHg, CI ≤ 2.5 L.min^{-1}.m^{-2}	Combined primary: proportion with ≥ 30% increase in cardiac output ≥ 25% reduction in PCWP at 24 hours Secondary: mortality	Primary end point: Levosimendan 28% vs. dobutamine 15% ($p = 0.022$) Secondary end points: mortality at 31 days – Levosimendan 8% vs. dobutamine 17% ($p = 0.049$) Mortality at 180 days: Levosimendan 26% vs. dobutamine 38% ($p = 0.029$)
RUSSLAN (2002) ($n = 504$)	Randomised, placebo controlled, double-blind	Levosimendan: Group 1 (G1): 6 mcg.kg^{-1} + 0.1 mcg.kg^{-1}.min^{-1} Group 2 (G2): 12 mcg.kg^{-1} + 0.2 mcg.kg^{-1}.min^{-1} Group 3 (G3): 24 mcg.kg^{-1} + 0.2 mcg.kg^{-1}.min^{-1} Group 4 (G4): 24 mcg.kg^{-1} + 0.4 mcg.kg^{-1}.min^{-1} Placebo	MI complicated by HF within last five days; HF on chest radiograph; systolic BP > 90 mmHg	Combined primary: proportion with hypotension or ischaemia at six hours Secondary: death or worsening HF at 24 hours Mortality at 180 days	Hypotension or ischaemia G1: 10.7%, G2: 12%, G3: 12.1%, G4: 19% Placebo: 10.8% ($p = 0.456$) Death or worsening of HF at 24 hours – G1: 5.8%, G2: 3%, G3: 3%, G4: 4% Placebo: 8.8% ($p = 0.089$) Mortality at 180 days G1: 26.2%, G2: 16%, G3: 27.3%, G4: 21% Placebo: 31.4% ($p = 0.088$)
REVIVE I (2004) ($n = 100$)	Randomised, placebo-controlled	24-hour infusion of levosimendan vs. placebo	Acute decompensated heart failure, dyspnoea at rest, unresponsive to iv diuretics	Global outcomes at five days	Improvement: Levosimendan 51% vs. placebo 33% Worsening: Levosimendan 20% vs. placebo 35% (overall $p = 0.043$)

Trial	Study design	Treatment	Population	Primary endpoint	Results
CASINO (2004) ($n = 227$)	Randomised, placebo-controlled, double-blind	Levosimendan vs. dobutamine vs. placebo for 24-hour infusion (doses not available from abstract)	NYHA IV EF $\leq 35\%$	Primary: combined death or re-hospitalisation owing to deterioration of HF	Levosimendan 30.6% vs. dobutamine 52.7% vs. placebo 48.1% (overall $p = 0.01$)
SURVIVE (2005) ($n = 1327$)	Randomised, double-blind	Levosimendan: 12 mcg.kg^{-1} bolus + 0.1–0.2 mcg.kg^{-1}.min^{-1} for 24 hours Dobutamine: 5 mcg.kg^{-1}.min^{-1}	Acute decompensated heart failure (EF $\leq 30\%$) requiring inotropic support owing to an insufficient response to iv diuretics and/or vasodilators	Primary: all-cause mortality at 5, 14, 28 and 180 days	Mortality reduced by 27%, 14%, 13%, 6.4% respectively ($p =$ NS)
REVIVE II (2005) ($n = 600$)	Randomised, placebo controlled, double-blind	Levosimendan: 6 or 12 mcg.kg^{-1} bolus + 0.1–0.2 mcg.kg^{-1}.min^{-1} for 24 hours Placebo	Acute decompensated heart failure, dyspnoea at rest despite iv diuretics, EF $\leq 35\%$	Primary: composite end point at five days	Improvement: Levosimendan 19.4% vs. placebo 14.6% Worsened: Levosimendan 19.4% vs. placebo 27.2% ($p = 0.015$)

BP = blood pressure; EF = ejection fraction; HF = heart failure; MI = myocardial infarction; NYHA = New York Heart Association; NS = non-significant; PCWP = Pulmonary artery wedge pressure.

subjects receiving β-blockers. Using β-blockers attenuated the inotropic and vasodilator effects in the dobutamine group, but not in the levosimendan group. Based on the sub-group analysis, levosimendan appears to be a superior choice in patients receiving concomitant β-blockers.

The RUSSLAN study

The RUSSLAN study (randomised study on safety and effectiveness of levosimendan in patients with left ventricular failure after an acute myocardial infarction) showed outcome benefits in comparison with placebo.[17] The study, which was conducted in Russia and Latvia, used safety as the primary outcome measure. Five hundred and four patients with decompensated heart failure following an acute myocardial infarction were randomised to receive one of four different doses of levosimendan or placebo. Levosimendan was administered as a loading dose of 6, 12, 24 or 24 mcg.kg^{-1} followed by a six-hour infusion of 0.1, 0.2, 0.2 or 0.4 mcg.kg^{-1}. min^{-1} respectively. During the first 24 hours there was a significant, dose-related decrease in the combined risk of worsening heart failure or death in patients treated with levosimendan (4.0% vs. 8.8% in the placebo group ($p = 0.044$)).

Mortality at 14 days was 11.7% for the combined levosimendan groups and 19.6% in the placebo group ($p = 0.031$); however, there was no difference at 180 days. There was no significant difference in the percentage of patients with combined hypotension and/or ischaemia in the levosimendan group.

The REVIVE I study

REVIVE I was a placebo-controlled pilot study assessing global outcomes (improved or worsening heart failure).[18] Worsening heart failure was defined as the need for intravenous vasodilators, inotropes or diuretics. More levosimendan patients improved and fewer experienced worsening heart failure than those administered placebo (overall $p = 0.043$). Subjects in the levosimendan treatment arm had a mean reduction of one day in the length of intensive care unit and hospital stay.

The CASINO study

The CASINO study has yet to be published; however, results were presented at the 53rd Annual Scientific Session of the American College of Cardiology.[19] This was a study comparing levosimendan to either placebo or dobutamine. The abstract reported that the primary end point was the combination of mortality or rehospitalisation for worsening heart failure. The levosimendan group (30.6%) had significantly better outcomes compared with placebo (48.1%) and dobutamine (52.7%) groups ($p = 0.01$). An interim analysis showed superiority of levosimendan over dobutamine and placebo and the trial was consequently stopped.

The SURVIVE study

The Survival of patients with acute heart failure in need of Intravenous inotropic support study (SURVIVE) was the first large-scale mortality trial comparing levosimendan and dobutamine in patients with acute decompensated heart failure.[20] This study has been presented and published in abstract form but has not yet been peer reviewed.

SURVIVE was a randomised, double-blind, double-dummy trial study carried out in 1327 patients enrolled at 75 sites in nine countries (Europe and Israel). All patients were hospitalised for acute decompensated heart failure and had a left ventricular ejection fraction of $\leq 30\%$, measured within 12 months before the start of the trial. Patients required intravenous inotropic therapy because of an insufficient response to intravenous diuretics and/or vasodilators, with oliguria and/or dyspnoea at rest. Patients were randomised to receive either a bolus of levosimendan ($12\,\mathrm{mcg.kg^{-1}}$) followed by a stepped dose regimen of levosimendan ($0.1\text{--}0.2\,\mathrm{mcg.kg^{-1}.min^{-1}}$) or dobutamine (minimum dose $5\,\mathrm{mcg.kg^{-1}.min^{-1}}$). Levosimendan was infused for a maximum of 24 hours, while dobutamine could be continued beyond 24 hours if thought clinically necessary. Both treatment groups also received standard of care.

The primary end point, 180-day all-cause mortality, did not differ significantly between the two treatment arms ($p = 0.401$). A secondary end point, β-type natriuretic peptide (BNP), was significantly reduced in the levosimendan arm compared with the dobutamine arm. The BNP levels were equally high in both groups at baseline, but after five days of treatment, BNP decreased by 46% in those who received levosimendan compared to 13% in the dobutamine group. Other secondary end points including days alive out of hospital during 180 days, change in dyspnoea and patient global assessment at 24 hours, and 180-day cardiovascular mortality were similar in both treatment arms.

The REVIVE II study

The second Randomised multicentre Evaluation of Intravenous levosimendan Efficacy (REVIVE II) study showed that patients who received levosimendan in addition to standard therapy were more likely to show clinical improvement and less likely to deteriorate than patients on standard therapy alone.[21] The REVIVE II study was the first large, prospective, randomised, double-blind, controlled trial to compare the effects of levosimendan plus standard therapy with the effects of standard therapy alone. Standard therapy consisted of diuretics, vasodilators and inotropes. The study was therefore designed to assess clinical practice, where multiple agents are used in combination. This study has been presented and published in abstract form but has not yet been peer reviewed.

Six hundred patients were recruited into this study at 103 sites in the United States, Australia and Israel. The mean age was 63 years and 73% of patients were male. All patients had been hospitalised for worsening heart failure and had dyspnoea at rest, despite treatment with intravenous diuretics, and a left ejection fraction of $\leq 35\%$ measured within the last year.

The primary end point of the study was a new clinical composite end point derived from studies in chronic heart failure and was first evaluated in REVIVE I. The end point consisted of a combination of patients' self-assessed symptoms together with a physician's assessment of the occurrence of clinical deterioration. The three-stage end point consisted of a ranking of:

1. Improved: moderately or markedly improved patient global assessment at six hours, 24 hours and five days with no worsening)
2. Unchanged: neither improved nor worse
3. Worse: death from any cause, persistent or worsening heart failure requiring intravenous medications (diuretics, vasodilators or inotropes) at any time, or moderately or markedly worse patient global assessment at six hours, 24 hours or five days.

Five days was selected as that was the average time a patient with acute decompensated heart failure spends in hospital. Patients were randomised to receive either a levosimendan bolus (6–12 mcg.kg^{-1}) followed by a stepped dose regimen of levosimendan (0.1–0.2 mcg.kg^{-1}.min^{-1}) for 24 hours plus standard therapy, or a placebo infusion for 24 hours plus standard therapy. Observations were continued for four days after the continuation of treatment.

After five days, more patients receiving levosimendan experienced improvement compared to those who were on placebo (19.4% vs. 14.6% respectively, a 33% relative increase; $p = 0.015$). Fewer patients receiving levosimendan worsened compared to patients who were on placebo (19.4% vs. 27.2% respectively), a 29% relative decrease. Fewer patients receiving levosimendan required rescue therapy (15.1% vs. placebo

Table 8.2 Adverse effects.

	SURVIVE		REVIVE II	
	Levosimendan	Dobutamine	Levosimendan	Placebo
Hypotension	15.5%	13.9%	50%	36%
Ventricular tachycardia	7.9%	7.3%	25%	17%
Atrial fibrillation	9.1%	6.1%	8%	2%
Cardiac failure	12.3%	17.0%	23%	27%

26.2%), a 42% relative decrease. The percentage of patients who did not meet the criteria for improvement or worsening was comparable in the two groups (61% for levosimendan vs. 58 % for placebo).

Secondary end points included β natriuretic peptide (BNP) levels and length of hospital stay. At 24 hours, BNP was significantly decreased in the levosimendan arm compared to the placebo and patients in the levosimendan group also experienced a shorter length of stay than the placebo group (7.0 days vs. 8.9 days respectively, $p = 0.001$). Other secondary end points, including patient global assessment and dyspnoea at six hours, were also significantly improved in the levosimendan arm. The incidence of adverse effects associated with levosimendan are outlined in Table 8.2.

The REVIVE II study was not primarily designed or powered to assess mortality. A secondary end point of mortality at 90 days did not differ significantly between treatment arms, although there were more deaths in the levosimendan arm (35 deaths vs. 45 deaths).

Interactions with other medicines

Levosimendan has been used safely with other cardiovascular drugs. Concurrent use of angiotensin-converting enzyme inhibitors, β-blockers and nitrates does not affect the positive inotropic effects of levosimendan.[22,23,24] Plasma protein binding and measures of coagulation were largely unaffected when oral levosimendan was administered with warfarin. The half-life of warfarin was significantly shorter and the volume of distribution was increased during co-administration with levosimendan.[25,26]

There is limited published information on pharmacokinetic drug interactions involving the hepatic cytochrome P 450 system. One study evaluated itraconazole, a CYP3A4 enzyme inhibitor. This study found no evidence of an interaction between itraconazole 200 mg and a single oral dose of levosimendan 2 mg in 12 healthy volunteers.[27]

Conclusion

Levosimendan is a novel and extremely interesting agent. It is the first inotropic drug ever to show outcome improvement against placebo for the treatment of acute heart failure. Unfortunately the mortality reduction demonstrated in early studies has not been borne out in the larger multi-centred protocols. Whether this is a real finding or an artefact of trial design is a little unclear. However the drug did lead to symptom improvement and shortened hospital stay, therefore justifying its use. An area of particular interest is the suggestion that it may be beneficial when compared against dobutamine. Dobutamine is the standard choice inotrope for this class of patients. If the findings show that levosimendan is superior to dobutamine, then a major shift in clinical practice would be justified. Unfortunately the SURVIVE study did not confirm these findings.

Levosimendan therefore represents the first drug in a new class of agents. It is an attractive therapeutic agent as it exerts a positive inotropic effect without increasing myocardial oxygen demand. Early data suggest that it is beneficial when compared to both placebo and dobutamine in terms of symptom relief and improvement in major outcome markers. If the early data are confirmed, then levosimendan would represent a significant advance on current therapies for the treatment of severe acute heart failure.

References

1. Ng TMH. Levosimendan, a new calcium-sensitizing inotrope for heart failure. *Pharmacotherapy* 2004; **24**: 1366–84.
2. Sorsa T, Heikkinen S, Abbott MB, *et al*. Binding of levosimendan, a calcium sensitiser, to cardiac troponin C. *J Biol Chem* 2001; **276**: 9337–43.
3. McBride BF, White CM. Levosimendan: implications for clinicians. *J Clin Pharmacol* 2003; **43**: 1071–81.
4. Brixius K, Reicke S, Schwinger RHG. Beneficial effects of the Ca^{2+} sensitizer levosimendan in human myocardium. *Am J Physiol Heart Circ Physiol* 2002; **282**: H131–7.
5. Hasenfuss G, Pieske B, Castell M, *et al*. Influence of the novel inotropic agent levosimendan on isometric tension and calcium cycling in failing human myocardium. *Circulation* 1998; **98**: 2141–7.
6. Haikala H, Kaheinen P, Levijoki J, Linden IB. The role of cAMP- and cGMP-dependent protein kinases in the cardiac actions of the new calcium sensitizer, levosimendan. *Cardiovasc Res* 1997; **34**: 536–46.
7. Ajiro Y, Hagiwara N, Katsube Y, Sperelakis N, Kasanuki H. Levosimendan increases L-type Ca^{2+} current via phosphodiesterase-3 inhibition in human cardiac monocytes. *Eur J Pharmacol* 1997; **333**: 249–59.
8. Janssen PM, Datz N, Zeitz O, Hasenfuss G. Levosimendan improves diastolic and systolic function in failing human myocardium. *Eur J Pharmacol* 2000; **404**: 191–9.

9. Yokoshiki H, Katsube Y, Sunagawa M, Sperelakis N. Levosimendan, a novel Ca^{2+} sensitizer, activates the glibenclamide-sensitive K^+ channels in rat arterial monocytes. *Eur J Pharmacol* 1997; **333**: 249–59.

10. Michaels AD, McKeown B, Kostal M, *et al*. Effects of intravenous levosimendan on human coronary vasomotor regulation, left ventricular wall stress, and myocardial oxygen uptake. *Circulation* 2005; **111**: 1504–9.

11. Jonsson EN, Antila S, McFadyen L, Lehtonen L, Karlsson MO. Population pharmacokinetics of levosimendan in patients with congestive heart failure. *Br J Clin Pharmacol* 2004; **57**: 412–15.

12. Kivikko M, Antila S, Eha J, Lehtonen L, Pentikainen PJ. Pharmacodynamics and safety of a new calcium sensitizer, levosimendan, and its metabolites during an extended infusion in patients with severe heart failure. *J Clin Pharmacol* 2002; **42**: 43–51.

13. Figgitt DP, Gillies PS, Goa KL. Levosimendan. *Drugs* 2001; **61**: 613–27.

14. Jonsson EN, Antila S, McFayden L, Lehtonen L, Karlsson MO. Population pharmacokinetics of levosimendan in patients with congestive heart failure. *Br J Clin Pharmacol* 2003; **55**: 544–51.

15. Antila S, Kivikko M, Lehtonen L, *et al*. Pharmacokinetics of levosimendan and its circulating metabolites in patients with heart failure after an extended continuous infusion of levosimendan. *Br J Clin Pharmacol* 2004; **57**: 412–15.

16. Follath F, Cleland JG, Just H, *et al*. Steering Committee and Investigators of the Levosimendan Infusion versus Dobutamine (LIDO) Study. Efficacy and safety of intravenous levosimendan compared to dobutamine in severe low-output heart failure (the LIDO study): a randomised double-blind trial. *Lancet* 2002; **360**: 196–202.

17. Moiseyev VS, Poder P, Andrejevs N, *et al*. RUSSLAN Study Investigators. Safety and efficacy of a novel calcium sensitizer, levosimendan, in patients with left ventricular failure due to an acute myocardial infarction. A randomized, placebo-controlled, double-blind study (RUSSLAN). *Eur Heart J* 2002; **23**: 1422–32.

18. Johansson S, Apajaslo M, Sarapohja T, Garratt C. Effect of levosimendan treatment on length of hospital and intensive care stay in the REVIVE I study (abstract). Presented at: 24th International Symposium on Intensive Care and Emergency Medicine, Mar 20–Apr 2, 2004, Brussels, Belgium. http://ccforum.com/content/8/S1/P88.

19. Zairis MN, Apostolatos C, Anastasiadis P, *et al*. The effect of the calcium sensitizer or an inotrope or none in chronic low-output decompensated heart failure: results from the Calcium Sensitizer or Inotrope or None in Low Output Heart Failure study (CASINO) (abstract). *J Am Coll Cardiol* 2004; **43** (Suppl 1): A206–7.

20. Mebazaa A, Cohen-Solal A, Kleber F, *et al*. Study design of a mortality trial with intravenous levosimendan (the SURVIVE study) in patients with acutely decompensated heart failure. *Crit Care* 2004; **8** (Suppl 1): P87.

21. Packer M. REVIVE II: Multicentre placebo-controlled trial of levosimendan on clinical status in acutely decompensated heart failure. Program and abstracts from the American Heart Association Scientific Sessions 2005; November 13–16, 2005 Dallas, Texas. Late Breaking Clinical Trials II.

22. Lehtonen L, Sundberg S. The contractility enhancing effect of the calcium sensitizer levosimendan is not attenuated by carvidelol in healthy subjects. *Eur J Clin Pharmacol* 2002; **58**: 449–52.

23. Antila S, Eha J, Heinpalu M, *et al.* Haemodynamic interactions of a new calcium sensitizing drug levosimendan and captopril. *Eur J Clin Pharmacol* 1996; **49**: 451–8.
24. Sundberg S, Lehtonen L. Haemodynamic interactions between the novel calcium sensitizer levosimendan and isosorbide-5-mononitrate in healthy subjects. *Br J Clin Pharmacol* 2000; **55**: 793–9.
25. Antila S, Järvinen A, Honkanen T, *et al.* Pharmacokinetic and pharmacodynamic interactions between the novel calcium sensitizer levosimendan and warfarin. *Eur J Clin Pharmacol* 2000; **56**: 705–10.
26. Antila S, Järvinen A, Honkanen T, *et al.* A new calcium sensitizing agent levosimendan has no pharmacokinetic or pharmacodynamics interaction with warfarin (abstract no. 382). *Eur J Clin Pharmacol* 1997; **52**: Suppl A128.
27. Antila S, Honkanen T, Lehtonen L, Neuvonen PJ. The CYP3A4 inhibitor intraconazole does not affect the pharmacokinetics of a new calcium-sensitizing drug levosimendan. *Int J Clin Pharmacol Ther* 1998; **36**: 446–9.

Lesley Durham and Brian H. Cuthbertson

Critical care outreach: six years on

It has been nearly six years since 'Comprehensive Critical Care' heralded the introduction of Critical Care Outreach services in England.[1] Whilst still the source of much critical debate, Critical Care Outreach has been, and remains, a central feature of recent approaches to address capacity pressures, and the management of the ever increasing numbers of acutely unwell and critically ill patients in National Health Service (NHS) hospitals regardless of their location – the oft cited 'Critical Care without Walls' approach.

Context and background of critical care outreach

Critical and acute care provision in England has changed drastically over the last 20 years. Between 1982 and 1995 there was a 25% decrease in the number of acute hospital beds. At the same time the population has grown and demand increased. The provision of critical care is made more difficult in the UK by factors such as low levels of staffing compared to other developed countries, an ageing population, the availability of increasingly complex clinical procedures, the increasing number of patients requiring Level 1 care in general wards, increased public awareness and expectation, changes in nursing education and staffing, changes in medical education and work practices including the new consultant contract, European Working Time Directive and Modernising Medical Careers. This has led to an inadequate provision of critical care beds.[2]

For many years clinical intuition, clinical experience and anecdotal evidence have suggested that care offered to patients in the period preceding

Recent Advances in Anaesthesia and Intensive Care 24, ed. J. N. Cashman and R. M. Grounds.
Published by Cambridge University Press. © Cambridge University Press 2007.

transfer to the intensive care unit (ICU) is often inadequate. There is now much published literature to support this claim, namely that: adverse events in hospitals associated with inadequate medical and nursing management are frequent,[3,4,5,6,7] unexpected cardiac arrests in hospital are usually preceded by signs of clinical instability for many hours,[8,9] and there is sub-optimal management both of patients discharged from ICU and of patients at risk of deterioration on the wards.[10,11] McQuillan and colleagues found that up to 41% of ward patients were transferred to critical care too late to achieve significant improvement in patient outcome.[5] Their research concluded that patient management was sub-optimal and that this had led to increased morbidity and mortality.

In answer to some of these issues 'comprehensive critical care' recognised that intensivists should become involved in the care of critically ill patients wherever they are located throughout the hospital.[1] This has been described as 'critical care without walls'. The same document also gave a 'high priority' recommendation that critical care outreach services and early warning scoring systems should be introduced in hospitals throughout England in order to address some of the shortfalls in patient care and outcomes identified and discussed above.

In response to the comprehensive critical care review the medical profession has produced position statements and guidance on the development of out-reach critical care. The Intensive Care Society (ICS) published 'Guidelines for the Introduction of Outreach Services – Standards and Guidelines in 2002'.[12] This document gives detailed clinical guidance, and also guidance on the membership of outreach teams, education, initiation of service and on audit and research. The Royal College of Physicians (RCP) produced a position statement entitled 'Three Ways to Improve Care for Seriously Ill Patients,' also in 2002.[13] It recognised that the organisation of care for acutely ill patients must change. In a further document the 'Interface between Acute General Medicine and Critical Care', the RCP working party made a number of recommendations that put the seriously ill patient at the centre of the service.[14] Better organisation of services would include the introduction of early warning scoring systems and of outreach services. Additionally, critical care outreach services have been advocated by the NHS Modernisation Agency,[15] NCEPOD[6,7], and latterly the Critical Care Stakeholders Forum.[16] Further, the NCEPOD document 'An Acute Problem' recommended outreach services and 'track and trigger' (TT) systems in their report.[17] This was despite the fact that their report highlighted major problems with medical acute care management even in the presence of outreach and TT in the majority of study hospitals. Yet investment in critical care outreach remains variable, and the service poorly developed in some organisations.[16]

Global models of critical care outreach

The terms medical emergency teams, rapid response teams, patient at risk teams and critical care outreach teams or 'Outreach' are used analogously, but in fact have some distinct differences.

The medical emergency team

The outreach concept originated in Liverpool, New South Wales, Australia in 1990 with the development of the medical emergency team (MET)[18]. The MET was developed in an effort to reduce the incidence of and improve outcome from cardiopulmonary arrests, by a doctor-led multidisciplinary team, modelled on the principles of early recognition and rapid response. The MET replaced the traditional cardiac arrest team with a more pro-active team of critical care doctors and nurses who would use a specified calling system to allow them to recognise impending critical illness and to intervene early to improve outcome.

The rapid response team

A rapid response (RR) team is a team of clinicians who bring critical care expertise to the patient bedside and is the model adopted in the USA. The Institute of Heath Improvement's review of literature and members' experience (2004) revealed that there were three main systemic issues in the USA that contributed to the problem: failures in planning, failure to communicate and failure to recognise deteriorating patient condition.[19,20] These fundamental problems which, on analysis, appear to be global, often lead to a 'failure to rescue'. Proponents of RR teams claim that establishing such teams will positively impact on the situation described above, by identifying unstable patients and those patients likely to suffer cardiac or respiratory arrest.

The patient at risk team

The UK critical care outreach model has evolved over the last nine years from the original concept of the 'patient at risk' (PAR) team introduced in 1997.[21] It differs from the Australian MET model in the way expert assistance is summoned. In this model a combination of predefined physiological criteria is used to assist ward nurses in identifying patient problems early on, calling a doctor and instituting prescribed therapy. If the ward nurses failed to get an adequate response from the doctor, then the PAR team was contacted to provide rapid intervention.[21]

The critical care outreach team

The function of these teams has not been confined only to the active treatment of patients for whom critical care would be beneficial. There has been discussion on the roles of PAR teams and METs in identifying patients for whom resuscitation would be inappropriate. By taking an active role in decisions to designate patients as "do not attempt to resuscitate" (DNAR) or 'not for ICU', these teams will undoubtedly contribute to lowering the incidents of inappropriate cardiopulmonary resuscitation with a consequent beneficial effect on the use of critical care resources.[21] However, some have said that the important end focus to be maintained is the overall improvement in care for the patient rather than purely a reduction in the incidents of cardiac arrest.

Objectives of the critical care outreach team

The National Outreach Forum defines critical care outreach as 'an organisational approach to ensure equity of care for all critically ill patients irrespective of their geographical location'. Critical care outreach is best explained as a systems approach for identifying and managing patients at risk of critical illness through collaborative care and education.[22] This model is predominantly nurse led, and tries to adopt a facilitative, empowering and supportive approach.

Since the publication of 'Comprehensive Critical Care', the ICS has expanded the original objectives of outreach. The five main aims for outreach services as specified by the ICS are:

- To avert (unnecessary) admissions to critical care

- To facilitate timely admissions to critical care and discharges to the ward

- To share critical care skills and expertise through educational partnerships

- To promote continuity of care

- To ensure thorough audit and evaluation of outreach services

These objectives are supported by the notion that critical care outreach should be a collaboration and partnership between the ICU and ward-based teams. It is further suggested that this is one of the reasons that this model has been not only accepted but also embraced, in spite of criticisms of a scant evidence base. Many critical care outreach teams have used these five objectives to demonstrate effectiveness at an organisational level with local audits and feedback. There seems little doubt that most critical care outreach teams are able to supply audit results demonstrating improvements in a variety of outcomes, and the feedback they receive demonstrates a subjective improvement in confidence in dealing with sick patients at the ward level. Of course this level of evidence rarely appears in the literature.

Components of critical care outreach

The National Outreach Forum (2003/6) recommends that the following are integral to critical care outreach services:

- Hospital-wide outreach available 24 hours a day
- Hospital wide track and trigger functions
- Outreach personnel free from other duties, appropriately skilled and trained to intervene
- Multiprofessional education and training function
- Follow-up functions after ICU discharge
- Research, audit, data collection functions
- Multiprofessional representation at Trust board level
- Public and patient involvement strategy

Early warning scoring and track and trigger systems

Integral to the British critical care outreach model are early warning scoring (EWS) systems or track and trigger (TT) systems. These systems have been developed to aid recognition of patient deterioration, but all lack validation. As yet there is no clear evidence identifying the ideal system. An EWS system can be described as 'a simple physiological scoring system with an identifiable trigger threshold'.[23] Early warning scoring systems are based upon the allocation of 'points' to physiological observations, the calculation of a total 'score' and the designation of an agreed calling 'trigger' level.[23,24,25,26] In all instances, when the trigger threshold is reached, in order for the system to work there needs to be a clear unambiguous referral pathway of expected actions and who is expected to perform these actions. This pathway should ideally form the basis of the critical care outreach operational policy and be ratified at hospital-wide level (see Tables 9.1 and 9.2).

Table 9.1 Classification of 'track and trigger' warning systems.

Single parameter systems
Tracking: periodic observation of selected basic vital signs
Trigger: one or more extreme observational values

Multiple parameter systems
Tracking: periodic observation of selected basic vital signs
Trigger: two or more extreme observational values

Aggregate weighted scoring systems
Tracking: periodic observation of selected basic vital signs and the assignment of weighted
    scores to physiological values with calculation of a total score
Trigger: achieving a previously agreed trigger threshold with the total score

Table 9.2 The early warning scoring system.[23]

Score	3	2	1	0	1	2	3
HR		<40	41–50	51–100	101–110	111–130	>131
Systolic BP	<70	71–80	81–100	101–199		>200	
Resp. rate		<8		9–14	14–20	21–29	>30
Temp(°C)		<35	35.1–36.5	36.6–37.4	>37.5		
CNS				A	V	P	U

Abbreviations – A = alert, V = responds to vocal stimuli, P = responds to painful stimuli,
U = unresponsive, HR = heart rate, BP = blood pressure, resp. rate = respiratory rate,
CNS = central nervous system score.

Skills, competencies and interventions of the critical care outreach team

The effectiveness of the decisions and actions taken by the critical care
outreach practitioner depends on the accuracy of the diagnosis, the ability
to recognise the presenting complaint(s) and underlying or associated pro-
blem(s), and the skills to intervene, in a context of the power and authority
to act.[26] As there exists a diversity of critical care outreach models, there
also exists diversity in the training and preparation undertaken by team
members, an issue currently being considered by National Outreach Forum
and the Critical Care Stakeholder Forum.

Multiprofessional educational programmes

One of the objectives of critical care outreach is to share critical care skills
and expertise through educational partnerships.[12] The Department of
Health also stated that 'high dependency care' training for ward staff should
be set up: 50% by March 2002, and 100% by 2004'. These 'targets' appear
to have dropped by the wayside, despite many critical care outreach teams
and practice based educators lobbying for the resources to meet them.

Nonetheless, there are an encouragingly large number of innovative multi-professional educational initiatives being delivered throughout the country: from health care assistant to 'refreshers' for medical consultants. Once again, many organisations have developed programmes with the fundamental goal that all staff providing acute care can recognise basic signs of deterioration and appreciate the necessity of obtaining timely and appropriate help.

Follow up after ICU discharge

Follow up after ICU is also offered by critical care outreach teams and can be divided into two distinct categories: follow up of all transfers out of ICU and follow up after hospital discharge. Robust follow up of transfers offers a number of advantages. Most importantly it provides reassurance and continuity of care for patients and their families, as both can feel a degree of anxiety when leaving the relative security and scrutiny of a designated Level 2 critical care area. Critical care outreach teams are able to support ward staff in the care and management of central lines, tracheostomies, chest drains, physiotherapy and nutritional regimes, all of which, it is suggested, may contribute to the prevention of avoidable ICU readmissions. Follow up after hospital discharge is not within the remit of this chapter.

Audit, evaluation and research

Despite a lack of resources, a great many critical care outreach teams have generated information about their services. In particular, frequency, nature and accuracy of vital observations, frequency of cardiac arrests, ICU re-admission rates, hospital length of stay, user satisfaction, prevalence of DNAR's, prevalence of EWS systems, identifying areas for targeted education, and the location of critical care needs within their hospitals. This process has been supported, and/or enabled by some networks in an attempt to evaluate organisational and regional critical care capacity requirements, with a view to informing commissioners. Sadly, to date, there remains little or no research capacity or funding in most critical care outreach teams. Whilst local audits have been used to demonstrate the effectiveness of critical care outreach teams at a local level, as yet they have not been analysed collectively, and many await the results of the NHS Research and Development Service Delivery and Organisation (SDO) Programme to inform future research and audit initiatives.

The current position

As suggested in the discussion above, with no central guidance or precise definition of what critical care outreach should look like, services have developed somewhat randomly. Team configuration and service delivery varies widely from single practitioners to multiprofessional models undertaking all component parts of critical care outreach. A recent unpublished national survey for the NHS Research and Development Service Delivery Organisation programme suggests that there are still a significant number of acute hospitals in England with no formal critical care outreach service. This result would seem to agree with the findings of NCEPOD's 'An Acute Problem'.[17] The data above suggest that the current position has changed little since the last National Survey undertaken by the National Outreach Forum in 2002. This survey also demonstrated that services varied widely in terms of team size and configuration, seniority and profession of service lead, hours of service provision, proportion of wards covered and interventions offered by the service. It could be argued that it is not desirable that there should be such variation in the operation of these teams or that perhaps these teams require to be custom designed to fit the hospital in which they are to function. However, the current situation is likely to continue until more evidence is available to guide clinical practice.

In relationship to frequency of vital observations, the authors would argue that all patients who are admitted to an acute care bed should 'routinely' have a track and trigger performed and recorded four hourly, with a clear unambiguous pathway of expected actions as a consequence of the track and trigger score. Of course in patients with physiological disturbance these observations must be performed more regularly. Evidence for sensitivity and specificity of these scores is lacking and a number of research projects are about to publish results in this area. There seems to be a suggestion that the scores lack sensitivity in a variety of clinical areas, perhaps suggesting that scoring systems require validation in all clinical areas and should not be used routinely across areas.[26] Durham and colleagues assert that 'one size does not fit all' and that local adjustment to the tool of choice is more important than the choice of tool.[27] It could be suggested that development of the definitive track and trigger has become the 'holy grail' of critical care outreach and track and trigger enthusiasts. Since critical care outreach teams depend on the sensitivity and specificity of the chosen track and trigger to allow early recognition and intervention, a score that lacks sensitivity will mean that these teams are unlikely to be efficacious or effective. Whatever your viewpoint, such a quest must be good for patients, as it has been the catalyst for much needed study into the role of abnormal physiology and scoring systems in identifying early deterioration in the ward patient.

Recent developments

An evaluation of outreach services in critical care

Given the diversity of critical care outreach models falling under the umbrella term of 'Outreach', in April 2003 the NHS Research and Development Service Delivery and Organisation Programme called for a rigorous scientific evaluation of critical care outreach services. The evaluation is taking a multicentre, multifaceted, multidisciplinary approach using different research designs. The study has been divided into seven sub-studies. This includes a systematic review of the literature on outreach services and early warning systems, a survey of outreach services in critical care, an interrupted time-series analysis and a multicentre, non-randomised study to evaluate the impact of critical care outreach services on patient outcomes from intensive care.

The care of the unexpectedly acutely ill patient in hospital

The Critical Care Stakeholder Forum (2006) has started a review of the care provided to patients on acute wards and in emergency departments, who are at risk of, or who ultimately go on to develop, critical illness. This work has been prompted by (among others) the NCEPOD report, and in recognition that the care of acutely ill patients could be improved. The proposed work will assume a three pronged approach:

(1) In collaboration with the National Institute for Clinical Excellence (NICE), clinical guidelines will be developed, inclusive of audit and implementation criteria.

(2) The identification of multiprofessional competencies, training needs and curriculum development undertaken by the Department of Health in collaboration with key stakeholder professional bodies and organisations.

(3) In collaboration with the National Outreach Forum, make more explicit the objectives, components, functions and standards that can be expected of critical care outreach.

These standards and objectives will then complement and interface with the clinical guidelines once developed. It is anticipated that draft guidelines will be available for comment in 2007.

Overview of the evidence

Calls for the justification of critical care outreach service provision are not new. Its value and the evidence to support its introduction have attracted criticism.[28] Most early work was performed in Australia. Buist and colleagues report a non-randomised, historically controlled study with a before-and-after design of the introduction of a MET into a teaching hospital.[29] The results demonstrate a decrease in the incidence of and mortality from unexpected cardiac arrests. This seems to be largely owing to the fact that they expected more cardiac arrests and placed more appropriate DNAR orders. The study also shows an increase in unplanned admissions to the intensive care unit after the introduction of the MET although the statistical significance of this is not stated. One problem raised by the authors was that the control and study periods were separated by some three years.[29] Bellomo and colleagues performed a prospective, controlled before-and-after trial to examine the effect of the introduction of an intensive care unit based medical emergency team in a large teaching hospital.[30] The team evaluated and treated any patient who was deemed to be at risk of developing an adverse outcome. The authors concluded that the introduction of the MET was associated with a significant reduction in the number of adverse events, postoperative mortality rate and mean duration of hospital stay. The authors note that the decrease in adverse events was only partly accounted for by the interventions of the MET and that the increased awareness of the significance and consequences of physiological instability lead to an improvement in care. The suggestion that education was an important factor seems to have been somewhat overlooked.

Bristow and colleagues published a prospective cohort comparison of three public hospitals.[31] At Hospital 1, the cardiac arrest team was replaced by a MET, at Hospitals 2 and 3, the arrest team operated as previously. Adjustment was made for case mix between hospitals. The results show that the MET hospital had fewer unanticipated ICU/HDU admissions mainly owing to the fact that they anticipated more of the admissions. However, there was no difference in either the in-hospital arrest rate or total death rate. In the UK, Leary and Ridley examined the effects of an outreach service on ICU readmissions to ICU, by comparing the numbers and reasons for readmission before and after the introduction of Outreach in their hospital.[32] They concluded that their study could detect no change in numbers or reasons for readmissions, and state that other parameters be used to examine the effectiveness of the outreach service, despite this being one of the highlighted aims of outreach.

Ball and colleagues published the results of a non-randomised population-based study, in which they compare historical controls with patients cared for by a nurse-only Outreach team, which was available for 12 hrs a day.[33] The team appears to have only seen patients who have been previously discharged from the ICU. They report that after the introduction of the outreach team there was a significant increase in survival to hospital discharge and a significant decrease in ICU readmission; however this decrease in readmission rate only returned the unit to the national average. Garcea and colleagues published a retrospective observational study, comparing before-and-after introduction of outreach covering surgical wards.[34] The team comprised two senior nurses and a nurse consultant and the service had an ICU consultant as the lead clinician, though their level of involvement is not defined. The team's remit involved the follow up of ICU/HDU discharges and education of ward staff with respect to the recognition of the sick patient; however this was later expanded to include the direct referral of patients highlighted by an early warning scoring system. They tentatively conclude that outreach teams may have a favourable impact on mortality rate among readmissions to critical care.

Preistly and colleagues performed a ward cluster randomised trial of phased introduction of critical care outreach to a general hospital.[35] A nurse consultant led their team, with a team of experienced nurses providing 24-hour cover. Ward staff used a locally devised patient-at-risk scoring system to trigger referral. This study found a significant reduction in hospital mortality in wards where the service operated compared to those where it did not. Analysis of whether outreach increased the length of hospital stay was equivocal, and data on cardiac arrest rate, overall hospital mortality, 'do not resuscitate' orders and ICU admissions are surprisingly not included. Importantly they also appear to demonstrate an improved outcome related to the pre-intervention educational programme. All these studies represent, at most, level 3 evidence and have major methodological weaknesses based on before-and-after designs, failure to use clear and important clinical end points and the high risk of bias associated with such designs including the Hawthorne effect (improving outcome by the process of observing or studying).

The MERIT study represents the best available evidence in the sphere of outreach and recruited 125 000 patients in 23 hospitals into a cluster randomised trial.[36] Australian hospitals with an ICU and emergency department that did not use the MET system were identified and offered the opportunity to participate in the study. The hospitals that agreed to participate were randomised to receive standardised MET implementation or to be controls and thus operate entirely as previously with no indication that a study was being undertaken. Over a period of four months an educational strategy was undertaken to prepare the study hospitals for the introduction of the MET; this included education of staff about calling criteria, identification of the patient at risk and the importance of rapidly calling the MET should any of the calling criteria be met. After MET implementation was complete an impressive system of reminders was continued to ensure that no calling criteria should be forgotten or overlooked. The study protocol required that the MET should be at least the equivalent of the pre-existing cardiac arrest team and should consist of at least one doctor and a nurse from the emergency department or ICU. The study results showed that the introduction of a MET system did not significantly reduce the incidence of any of the study outcomes (cardiac arrest, unexpected death or unplanned ICU admission). The authors, clearly disappointed by the negative result, pointed out three main flaws in their study's ability to disprove the null hypothesis. Firstly, they suggest that the six-month study period was inadequate as the study was underpowered. However, the very small difference in the incidence of the primary outcome measure between groups suggests that even if they did continue the study the number needed to treat to prevent a combined outcome would be approximately 2000. Hardly an effective intervention! Secondly, that in the control hospitals the cardiac arrest teams are often called to critically ill patients who have not suffered a cardiac arrest and thus are acting as informal METs. This is countered by the fact that far more MET calls were made in the intervention hospitals compared to control hospitals, although many calls were made inappropriately. The final point is that the study demonstrated a failure of the Hawthorne effect as even though the MET hospitals knew they were being studied the levels of monitoring, documentation and responses to changes in vital signs were grossly inadequate. They failed to comment on the fact that the trial demonstrated that the MET calling system failed to allow early recognition and intervention in their patients. This was evidenced by the fact that they failed to see half of the appropriate ICU admissions before their admission and failed to identify the majority of patients more than 15 minutes before an event. They also did not highlight the fact that the only significant improvement in outcomes in the trial was related to the pre-intervention educational programme. The finding that education could improve outcome from critical illness is indeed a major finding and should be given great emphasis. It would surely be far more cost-effective to educate staff than to provide 24-hour outreach cover. Countering this viewpoint, the National Outreach Forum argue that assertions that education alone will negate the need for 24-hour critical care outreach are shortsighted.

Conclusions

Critical care outreach services are generally considered one of the success stories of the modernisation of critical care, regardless of arguments on evidence base. Indeed latterly some of its fiercest opponents, who have observed first hand the contribution and benefits that collaboration and partnership with critical care outreach brings to their patients, have become supporters. There is arguably, however, a need to clarify and articulate with more precision, the components, role and boundaries of critical care outreach, and to make more explicit the standards of service that can be expected, inclusive of standardisation of the skills, competencies and interventions offered by critical care outreach teams, and to whom and where they are offered. Additionally, wider multiprofessional and cross-speciality collaboration and partnerships with the patients' needs firmly in the centre of decision-making will offer a more coherent approach, and thus result in a more efficient process and ultimately improve the quality of the patient experience and outcomes overall. Clearly education needs to be the cornerstone of future services and this can be performed at the bedside as well as in the large variety of excellent courses in the field of critical care. Finally, despite the increasing clinical support for outreach services and the subjective feeling that they are bringing about improvements in patient care, there is a need to develop an evidence base to support these claims and assure further funding and support.

References

1. UK Department of Health. *Comprehensive Critical Care. A Review of Adult Critical Care Services.* London: Department of Health, 2000.
2. Goldhill D, Mackinley A. Outreach critical care. *Anaesthesia* 2002; **57**: 183.
3. Brennan TA, Leap LL, Laird NM, *et al.* Incidents of adverse events and negligence in hospitalised patients: results of the Harvard Medical Practice study 1. *N Engl J Med* 1991; **324**: 370–6.
4. Wilson RM, Runciman WB, Gibberd RW, *et al.* The Quality in Australian Health Care Study. *Med J Aus* 1995; **163**: 458–71.
5. McQuillan P, Pilkington S, Allan A, *et al.* Confidential enquiry into quality of care before admission to intensive care. *BMJ* 1998; **316**: 1853–8.
6. The National Confidential Enquiry into Peri-operative Deaths 1996–97. *HMSO* 1997. Available online at: http://www.ncepod.org.uk/sum96.htm.
7. Scottish Audit of Surgical Mortality. Annual report 1996, SASM; Scotland 1997. Available online at: http://www.sasm.org.uk/Reports/2004Report/SASM_Report_2004_data.pdf.
8. Schein RMH, Hazday N, Pena M, Ruben BH, Sprung CL. Clinical antecedents to in-hospital cardiac arrest. *Chest* 1990; **98**: 1388–92.
9. Franklin C, Mathew J. Developing strategies to prevent in-hospital cardiac arrest: analysing responses of physicians and nurses in the hours before the event. *Crit Care Med* 1994; **22**: 244–7.
10. McGloin H, Adam SK, Singer M. Unexpected deaths and referrals to intensive care of patients on general wards. Are some cases potentially avoidable? *J R Coll Phys Lond* 1999; **33**: 255–9.
11. Goldhill DR, White SA, Sumner A. Physiological values and procedures in the 24 h before ICU admission from the ward. *Anaesthesia* 1999; **54**: 529–34.

12. Intensive Care Society. Guidelines for the introduction of outreach services 2002, http://www.ics.ac.uk/downloads/icsstandards-outreach.pdf.
13. http://www.rcplondon.ac.uk/.
14. Royal College of Physicians. The interface between Acute General Medicine and Critical Care 2002 http://www.rcplondon.ac.uk/pubs/ wp_ibagmacc_home.htm.
15. NHS Modernisation Agency. Critical care outreach 2003. http://www.modern. nhs.uk/scripts/default.asp?siteid=20.
16. Quality Critical Care: Beyond 'Comprehensive Critical Care': A report by the Critical Care Stakeholder Forum 2003. http://www.dh.gov.uk/ PublicationsAndStatistics/Publications/PublicationsPolicyAndGuidance/ PublicationsPolicyAndGuidanceArticle/fs/en?CONTENTID=4121049 &chk=C2CJv3.
17. An Acute Problem? The National Confidential Enquiry into Patient Outcome and Death. 2005 http://www.ncepod.org.uk/2005.htm.
18. Lee A, Bishop G, Hillman KM, Daffurn K. The medical emergency team. *Anaesth Intens Care* 1995; **23**: 183–6.
19. Institute of Health Improvement. Establish a rapid response team. 2006 http:// www.ihi.org/IHI/Topics/CriticalCare/IntensiveCare/Changes/ EstablishaRapidResponseTeam.htm.
20. Goldhill DR, Worthington L, Mulechy A, Tarling M, Sumner A. The patient-at-risk team: identifying and managing seriously ill ward patients. *Anaesthesia* 1999; **54**: 853–60.
21. Goldhill DR. Introducing the postoperative care team. *BMJ* 1997; **314**: 389.
22. Garrard C, Young JD. Sub-optimal care of patients before admission to intensive care. *BMJ* 1998; **316**: 1841–2.
23. Bright D, Walker W, Bion J. Clinical review: outreach – a strategy for improving the care of the acutely ill hospitalized patient. *Crit Care* 2004; **8**: 33–40.
24. Morgan RJM, Williams F, Wright MM. An early-warning scoring system for detecting developing critical illness. *Clin Intens Care* 1997; **8**: 100.
25. Stenhouse C et al. Prospective evaluation of modified EWS score. *Br J Anaesth* 2000; **84**: 663P.
26. Subbe CP, Kruger M, Rutherford P, Gemmel L. Validation of modified early warning score in medical admissions. *Q J Med* 2001; **94**: 521–6.
27. Durham L, Hancock H. Critical care outreach: an exploration of fundamental philosophy and underpinning knowledge. *Nurs Crit Care* 2006; **11**: 239–47.
28. Cuthbertson BH: Outreach critical care – cash for no questions? *Br J Anaesth* 2003; **90**: 4–6.
29. Buist M, Bernard S, Nguyen TV, Moore G, Anderson J. Association between clinically abnormal observations and subsequent in-hospital mortality: a prospective study. *Resuscitation* 2004; **62**: 137–41.
30. Bellomo R, Goldsmith D, Uchino S, *et al*. Prospective controlled trial of medical emergency team on postoperative morbidity and mortality rates. *Crit Care Med* 2004; **32**: 916–21.
31. Bristow PJ, Hillman TC, Chey T, *et al*. Rates of in-hospital arrests, deaths and intensive care admissions: the effect of a medical emergency team. *MJA* 2000; **173**: 236–40.
32. Leary T, Ridley S. Impact of an Outreach team on re-admissions to a critical care unit. *Anaesthesia* 2003; **58**: 328–32.

33. Ball C, Kirby K, Williams S. Effect of the critical care Outreach team on patient survival to discharge from hospital and readmission to critical care: non-randomised population based study. *BMJ* 2003; **327**: 1014–17.

34. Garcea G, Thomasset S, McClelland L, *et al*. Impact of a critical care Outreach team on critical care readmissions and mortality. *Acta Anaesth Scand* 2004; **48**: 1096–100.

35. Preistly G, Watson W, Rashidian A, *et al*. Introducing critical care Outreach: a ward-randomised trial of phased introduction in a general hospital. *Intensive Care Med* 2004; **30**: 1398–404.

36. Merit Study Investigators. Introduction of the medical emergency team (MET) system: a cluster randomised controlled trial. *Lancet* 2005; **365**: 2091–7.

Michael D. Christian, Thomas E. Stewart and
Stephen E. Lapinsky

CHAPTER

10

Critical care and biological disasters: lessons learned from SARS and pandemic influenza planning

Day to day, critical care units in Western society provide highly resourced intense care to patients with complex medical problems or injuries. Typically a relatively small number of patients are managed by highly educated and specialised physicians (intensivists) in collaboration with a large team of health care workers (HCWs), skilled specifically in dealing with critically ill patients including: critical care nurses, respiratory therapists, nutritionists, physiotherapists, pharmacists and other allied HCWs. Critical care is comprised of three core components: intensive nursing care with a 1:1 or 1:2 nurse-to-patient ratio, the provision of life support measures, and invasive monitoring including devices such as arterial lines or pulmonary artery catheters. Life support in this context can include ventilatory support with positive pressure mechanical ventilation, circulatory support with medications to control/support blood pressure (e.g. dopamine) or mechanical support (e.g. intra-aortic balloon pump or temporary transvenous pacemaker), and renal replacement therapy.

Whilst the model of care described above is effective for day-to-day patient management, during a disaster, particularly biological disasters, this model of care is often not sustainable nor an efficient use of limited resources.[1] The term biological disaster is used to refer to events such as infectious disease outbreaks (epidemics and pandemics) or bioterrorism attacks. This chapter will discuss issues related to providing critical care services during biological disasters including preparedness, organisational structure, communication, surge capacity, mass critical care, triage, infection control, and ethical challenges.

Severe acute respiratory syndrome (SARS)[2] acutely focused the attention of the world on the potential implications of biological disasters for

Recent Advances in Anaesthesia and Intensive Care 24, ed. J. N. Cashman and R. M. Grounds.
Published by Cambridge University Press. © Cambridge University Press 2007.

communities,[3,4] hospitals[5,6,7] and in particular critical care units.[8,9,10,11,12,13] Severe acute respiratory distress syndrome brought to fruition many of the concerns regarding bioterrorist attacks.[14] Although bioterrorism remains a threat, many feel that a pandemic of influenza is an equally pressing threat,[15,16,17] particularly with strains of H5N1 circulating in Asia and evidence of transmission to humans.[18,19] The three types of biological disasters discussed above (bioterrorism, epidemics and pandemics) share many common features and lessons.[20] However, the primary difference between these is the duration of the event. Bioterrorist attacks and epidemics tend to be relatively brief in duration (days to weeks), as opposed to pandemics that can last months to years.

Preparation

To prepare for a biological disaster, critical care units should (a) develop a plan, (b) train staff, and (c) exercise their plans and staff. It is critical that this planning not be done in isolation. The plan developed by critical care for their response to a biological disaster must be integrated with the broader hospital plan, that in turn should be part of a community-wide response plan.[21] Although much planning is done at a general level, plans regarding biological disasters, and in particular plans for specific departments such as critical care, need to include detailed operational plans for responses that may last up to 12–24 months in the case of a pandemic.[17] Extensive plans have been developed for managing an influenza pandemic. These include plans by governments ranging from the United Nations and federal governments, down to provincial, regional and municipal levels. In addition, many hospitals have also developed pandemic plans. Regardless of the level of planning, it is helpful if the structure of the planning committee mirrors the planned structure for the response. This makes it easier for those outside the planning process to connect with those involved in the process or find information they are searching for, as well as facilitating a transition to response should a pandemic occur.

Some authors identify staff education and training as the most important aspects of preparing to deal with biological disasters.[22] Education often must begin at the most basic level by increasing disaster awareness. Beyond the basics, critical care HCWs also need to understand their roles/responsibilities during a response, and develop disaster-specific skills such as infection control techniques and triage. Simulator training can be a valuable tool for training staff as well as testing plans (see Chapter 13).[9,22] Computer modelling may also be useful when planning for disasters, including biological disasters.[23,24,25]

Organisation and communication

Time and time again, prior disasters have identified the lack of a well-defined organisational structure with clear lines of command, control and communication as a key factor resulting in failures.[21,26,27] Unfortunately, despite this rich history, breakdowns in the organisational structure were also cited as a shortcoming during Toronto's response to SARS.[28,29] In response to similar issues the incident management system (IMS) was developed in the 1970s and has been widely used by various mobile first responders such as police, fire and emergency medical services (EMS).[21,26] The IMS is a tool for command, control and coordination of a response.[30] After nearly two decades, health care organisations and public health agencies have recently started to use IMS to structure their emergency responses.[31] In their article on lessons learned from SARS, Harwyluck and colleagues[9] describe the need for a critical care crisis team, the attributes of which could be fully met by implementing IMS. Although not a biological disaster, the New York University Downtown Hospital has identified the use of IMS as a critical factor in their ability to manage over 350 patients within the first two hours following the collapse of the World Trade Center.[32] This serves as a prime example of the utility of IMS for health care systems responding to disasters.

Critical care units should structure their response following the IMS model utilising objective focused task forces (e.g. care teams and resuscitation teams), with a clear chain of command and appropriate ratio of supervisors to team members between 1:5–1:7. The structure within the intensive care unit (ICU) would form a branch or division of the hospital's overall IMS response structure. One of the key benefits of using IMS is the standardisation of the nomenclature and organisation allowing outside agencies, such as public health, who are also using IMS, to easily interact with the health care system. The IMS also plays an important role in facilitating a hospital's surge response and triage activities.

The second major criticism of the SARS response in Toronto, and many prior disaster responses elsewhere, was poor communication.[9,28,29,33,34] A successful critical care response in a biological disaster requires good communication with both internal stakeholders (HCWs, administrators, unions, other departments) as well as with external stakeholders (outside agencies/organisations, patient family members, the public and press). Communication strategies should be incorporated into response plans and tested during exercises.

During SARS, although communication between groups such as public health, administration and front-line clinicians was suboptimal, individual groups (e.g. critical care, infectious diseases) developed effective communication strategies. One particularly useful communications strategy included regularly scheduled conference calls for physicians managing SARS patients.[33] These teleconferences allowed dissemination of infection control/treatment guidelines, co-ordinating data collection, rumour control and psychological support. Provincial and World Health Organisation-based secure web sites allowed the exchange of infection control and management protocols. Since biological disasters typically will involve more than one hospital, systems must be developed to allow easy networking and communication between critical care units within a region. The Greater New York Hospital Association has developed excellent examples of both radio and computerised communications networks. Further information can be obtained from their Emergency Preparedness Resource Center (http://www.gnyha.org/3/Default.aspx).

Surge response strategies

Given the current fiscal constraints on the health care system in both Canada and the USA, most ICUs operate at near 100% capacity on a day-to-day basis.[31] Therefore, even a minor biological disaster could easily overwhelm a hospital's critical care resources.[1] Plans and processes to deal with surges in patients related to biological disasters need to be included in a comprehensive emergency preparedness and management plan. Such plans employ various strategies depending on the magnitude of the situation (Fig. 10.1). Most ICUs are capable in dealing with small surges (i.e < 20–30% above their day-to-day capacity) without exceeding their ability to cope. However, larger demands on the system exceed a critical care unit's ability to respond and thus various strategies such as a code orange (disaster) response, mass critical care and ultimately 'TRUE (Targeting Response to Ultimate Ends) Triage' are required. Collectively these concepts are referred to as surge response strategies and will be discussed in further detail below.

Hick and colleagues[31] differentiate between two important concepts:

- Surge capacity: making available adequate resources to deal with increased number of patients

- Surge capability: ability to manage increased numbers of patients

These definitions illustrate the need to plan for staff resources in addition to equipment and facilities. For further information on surge capacity see Hicks' article[31] and web resources available at the Centre for Excellence in Emergency Preparedness (www.ceep.ca).

Response thresholds

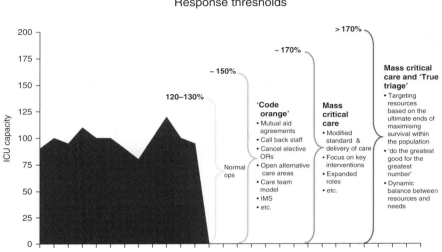

Fig. 10.1 The day-to-day capacity of most ICUs is near 100% utilisation. Response strategies to surges in demand caused by emergencies or disasters must be applied in a graded fashion depending on the predicted capacity represented by the brackets moving to the right in the diagram.

When considering options for rapidly expanding both critical care staff and facilities, two key considerations are (a) planning based on identifying functional requirements for managing critically ill patients and (b) maintaining up-to-date inventories of which staff or facilities meet the functional requirements. Table 10.1 lists the basic functional requirements that must be present for a critical care area. Examples of potential areas found in most hospitals that typically have such requirements without requiring modifications are listed in Table 10.2. Surge capacity should also be considered when designing new hospitals or during renovations. For example, hallways or large rooms such as cafeterias and physiotherapy rooms should have electrical outlets, oxygen, medical gas, and suction quick connects available behind removable panels to permit access in a disaster, thereby allowing these spaces to be reconfigured into critical care areas.

Another strategy to increase capacity is to modify the organisational structure in which care is provided through the use of care teams. In a care team a group of HCWs work together to care for a defined group of patients, usually in a fixed geographical area, in a pyramid supervisory structure with less educated staff being supervised and assisted by a small number of more skilled/experienced HCWs. This allows resources to be used more efficiently and for HCWs working in expanded roles to function safely and effectively. In the example provided in Fig. 10.2, typically six to eight ICU

Table 10.1 Functional requirements for providing critical care.

- Oxygen
- Suction
- Medical gas
- Electrical outlets
- Adequate space for equipment

Table 10.2 Potential environments for critical care surge.

- Medical ICU
- Surgical ICU
- CCU
- CVICU (Cardiovascular ICU)
- PACU (post-anaesthetic care unit/recovery room)
- Endoscopy units
- Day surgery
- Step-down units

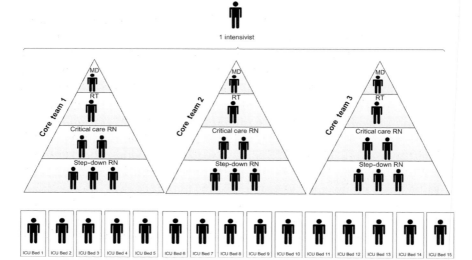

Fig. 10.2 In the care-team structure illustrated above, patients are cared for by teams of health care workers with varying levels of expertise and experience in critical care. Instead of having 1:1 ICU nurse:patient ratios, non-ICU nurses are incorporated into the structure, as are non-intensivist physicians to extend the human resources available.

RNs (registered nurses), 2 RTs (respiratory therapists) and 1 intensivist take care of ten ICU patients. Using care teams nine non-ICU RNs work with six ICU RNs, three RTs, three family physicians or junior residents and 1 intensivist to care for 15 critically ill patients. Using care teams a 50%

increase in the critical care human resources capacity could be obtained by supplementing experienced ICU staff with non-ICU staff. This structure is also consistent with the IMS organisational structure. Care teams were used in the emergency department during the September 11th response in New York with good results.[35] Similarly, ICU outreach teams for hospital wards and telephone support from academic intensivists for community intensivists may also be helpful to maintain system capacity.[33]

Typically a surge capacity strategy can increase a hospital's capacity by 20–30%.[31] However, rarely can critical care surge capacity exceed 10% owing to a combination of staff limitations and resource requirements. Most of the strategies outlined above and in the literature for surge capacity are oriented towards responding to short-term surges. As noted earlier in the chapter, surges associated with epidemics or pandemics tend to be prolonged compared to other biological disasters and non-biological disasters. For example, many predict that a pandemic of influenza will occur in multiple waves over the course of 12 to 24 months.[17] Thus, surge response strategies for a pandemic must consider both the magnitude and the duration of the surge.

The final factor to keep in mind when planning to respond to any surge, short or long, is organisational continuity. A single pool of health care resources exist that must be accessed by all. Thus, plans must be in place to provide care to those patients associated with the biological disaster as well as those with other medical/surgical issues. Patients will continue to have heart attacks, car accidents, give birth to babies and require hip replacements. Whilst resources may be scaled back to increase the capacity, provisions must exist to provide other essential services. During SARS, Toronto discovered the consequences of focusing only on a single issue and cancelling or severely curtailing all other services. After the two-month outbreak of SARS, the number of patients awaiting cardiac surgery increased by 15%, and completed cases decreased 40%. The long-term health consequences of such delays in health care services remain to be seen.[28,29,36] Although there is a need to ensure that other essential clinical services are provided during the biological disaster, the responsibility for ensuring this does not fall completely upon individual hospitals; regional planning and co-operation are necessary to ensure that within a geographic region all services are available somewhere. Similarly, during a pandemic or large infectious disease outbreak restrictions will be placed on the menu of laboratory testing available so that resources can be directed towards responding to the outbreak. Again however, it will be necessary to ensure that some laboratories continue to provide other non-pandemic related essential tests.

Mass critical care

When resource demands exceed even the 'typical' code-orange (disaster) surge capacity of a hospital, the next step is to institute mass critical care. Mass critical care is both a different model and a different standard of critical care from what is practised day to day. Simply stated, the goal of mass critical care is to provide a few key interventions (those with the highest impact and potential to save lives – see Table 10.3) to many people rather than providing very resource-intense interventions to a few.[1] All processes and procedures are open to modification and must be considered from a new perspective including standards of care, staffing, equipment and the allocation of resources. Decision-making should be objective-driven, consistent with the IMS model.[21,26]

A difficult but key decision is when to implement mass casualty critical care. One should not wait until resources are in scarce supply to make this decision. As soon as an emergency, in this case a biological disaster, is recognised the situation must be sized up, an estimate made of the potential casualty burden, and an accurate inventory of available resources compiled.[35] It is based upon the latter two factors that the decision whether to implement mass casualty critical care is made. If the predictions are that resource scarcities are going to occur, mass critical care strategies should be employed, beginning with the early influx of patients to optimise the use of available resources.[35] When managing biological disasters, however, the ability to conduct an accurate 'size-up' early in the emergency is difficult owing to challenges in recognising the occurrence of the event as well as predicting the possible magnitude.[37]

Table 10.3 Interventions in mass critical care.

High impact interventions
- Basic modes of ventilation
- Hemodynamic support
  - Fluid resuscitation
  - Basic inotropes (i.e. dopamine, norepinephrine)
- Antibiotics
- Disease-specific countermeasures
  - thrombolysis for myocardial infarctions
  - anti-toxin for bioterrorism agents
- Key prophylactic interventions
  - DVT prophylaxis
  - Ventilating patients with the head of the bed at 45°

Inefficient interventions
- Renal replacement therapy (e.g. dialysis)
- High-frequency oscillation ventilation
- Extracorporeal membrane oxygenation

Patient flow through the system is another key factor for success during a mass casualty response to a biological disaster. The flow of patients has implications for both the efficiency of care and infection control. The latter issue will be addressed more fully in the infection control section. During routine hospital care critically ill patients often enter through the emergency room (ER) where they are assessed. The patient may then go back and forth between the ER or ICU and several other departments such as surgery or radiology for various procedures and tests. This results in inefficient care and resource utilisation. During mass casualty critical care patients should only move through the system in a forward direction whenever possible (Fig. 10.3).

To further improve the efficiency of patient care the use of clinical pathways should be considered. Clinical pathways have been shown to improve patient care and decrease length of stay for patients with community acquired pneumonia.[38,39,40] Clinical pathways that include admission criteria, management protocols, infection-control protocols, and discharge criteria have several potential benefits. Such clinical pathways should be developed, in advance of a disaster when possible, for specific conditions (e.g. anthrax, small pox, hemorrhagic fevers, pandemic influenza, etc.). Firstly, in a large-scale emergency such as a pandemic, it will likely be necessary for health care workers to be working in expanded roles or in areas, such as ICU, other than where they typically work.[41,42] Well-constructed clinical pathways[41] will help provide guidance for management of patients whilst at the same time providing warning flags when patients are not responding appropriately, prompting expert assistance to be sought. Further, in order to maintain the integrity of the system, including critical care capacity, it is important to have a good flow of patients through the system. This can be facilitated by clear admission and discharge criteria.

Prior to leaving this topic, it is important to discuss the issue of altered standards of care during mass critical care. Although there certainly is a need to modify the standard of care compared to routine critical care during a biological disaster, one must always keep in mind the primary objective of trying to ensure that the maximum number of people possible survive. Thus, caution must be exercised when expanding clinical roles or modifying management to ensure that care is not compromised beyond the point where more harm is being done than good. For instance, it is of little use to move to a ventilation strategy that may allow many more people to be ventilated but in the end results in a significant increased number of deaths owing to barotrauma than would have occurred if fewer patients were ventilated using a less harmful ventilation strategy. Striking an appropriate

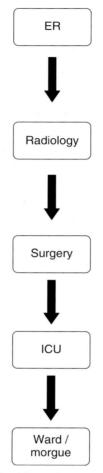

Fig. 10.3 Patient flow in a disaster should be unidirectional from one department to another. Not all patients must go to each department however. Patients not immediately requiring radiological investigations or surgery may go directly from the emergency department to the intensive care unit.

balance requires monitoring treatment outcomes during the response. Plans to alter the standard of care during mass critical care should be publically discussed and documented prior to any disaster, with clear and objective criteria for institution of mass critical care in order to comply to medico-legal and ethical standards.[43] For this same reason it is critical that all hospitals within an area adhere to the same standards of care.

'True' triage

During some biological disasters, surge capacity may be maximised and, despite the implementation of mass critical care, resource scarcities will still occur.[1] In such situations it is necessary, and in fact mandated by international law,[44,45,46] to utilise methods for allocating resources that are both equitable and maximise the benefit to the population at large.[31] Such methods can be referred to as 'triage' or 'TRUE' (Targeting Resources to Ultimate Ends) triage, not to be confused with the prioritisation 'triage' systems[47] used in emergency departments on a routine basis.[35] The original concept of 'triage' was developed during wartime[46] where scarce resources are used to provide the maximum benefit to the population at large, even if it means that individual victims who might have been saved under other circumstances cannot be treated optimally.[35,48]

Further, human rights, humanitarian laws[44] and strict adherence to ethical practices, such as transparency and accountability, must be observed when triage protocols are being developed.[1] Ethical values such as proportionality, equity and reciprocity necessitate a well thought out and co-ordinated approach to the allocation of scarce resources. Health care providers practising in a biological disaster have to balance the needs of individuals with the responsibility they also have to all others in the community as guardians of important resources. In short, the primary goal of triage during a biological disaster is to be able to 'do the greatest good, for the greatest number'.[35] A full exploration of the ethical issues related to triage can be found in the literature[45,46] as well as the framework developed by the Joint Centre for Bioethics.[43]

Prior to recent pandemic planning initiatives, no triage systems had been developed for use in critical care or medical illnesses. Illness severity scoring systems[49,50,51] currently used in critical care research have reasonable abilities to predict ICU outcome, but they are cumbersome to use and therefore particularly impractical for use during a biological disaster when human resources are scarce. Further, although validated for predicting outcome, they have not been validated for guiding, or more specifically restricting, treatment.

Christian and colleagues have recently published the first comprehensive triage protocol designed for use during a pandemic as well as potential applicability to other large disasters.[52] This protocol has been incorporated into the Ontario Pandemic Influenza Plan.[41] The triage protocol utilises the Sequential Organ Failure Assessment score[53] and has four main components: inclusion criteria, exclusion criteria, minimum qualifications for survival, and a prioritisation tool (Fig. 10.4).

Military triage systems[54,55,56] are good only as a model for critical care triage during biological disasters since they were devised specifically for

Colour code	Initial assessment	48-hour assessment	120-hour assessment	Priority/Action
Blue	Exclusion criteria* or SOFA > 11*	Exclusion criteria or SOFA > 11 or SOFA 8–11 no Δ	Exclusion criteria* or SOFA > 11* or SOFA < 8 no Δ	Medical Mgmt +/– Palliate & d/c from CC
Red	SOFA ≤ 7 or Single organ failure	SOFA score < 11 and decreasing	SOFA score < 11 and decreasing progressively	Highest
Yellow	SOFA 8–11	SOFA < 8 no Δ	SOFA < 8 with < 3-point decrease in past 72 h	Intermediate
Green	No significant organ failure	No longer ventilator dependent	No longer ventilator dependent	Defer or d/c, reassess as needed

Fig. 10.4 The prioritisation tool for use in the critical care triage protocol.
*If exclusion criteria or SOFA > 11 occurs at any time from initial assessment to 48 hours, change triage code to blue and palliate; CC = critical care; d/c = discharge; Δ = change; SOFA = Sequential Organ Failure Assessment Score.
Source: Adapted from: Christian et al.[52]

trauma and not medical conditions or biological events. The 'SEIRV' triage system was developed for use in bioterrorism attacks and is used to categorise patients as susceptible, exposed, infectious, removed and vaccinated (SEIRV).[37] Although a very robust system which provides many lessons that can and should be applied to the overall response to biological disasters, it does not address issues dealing with resource allocation. The SEIRV system uses inclusion, exclusion and minimum qualifications for survival (MQS) to guide triage decisions. These should also be used in all critical care triage systems.

A significant challenge in developing critical care triage protocols for biological disasters is that often prior to a biological disaster multiple unknown factors exist including the nature of the biological disaster, the natural history and prognostic indicators. An additional layer of complexity is added to this equation when one also recognises that the triage of critical care resources during a biological disaster applies not only to victims of the biological disaster, but also to all patients who require critical care resources for other reasons. Given the highly complex nature of the system and processes that must be developed, it is impossible to create such a system from scratch during the middle of a biological disaster.[1]

The best way to prepare for critical care triage during a biological disaster is to develop general baseline triage guidelines[52] in advance of a biological disaster and then modify the protocol once variable factors such as probability of survival and available resources are known. Another area where

Table 10.4 Key triage infrastructure development initiatives.

1. The availability of accurate and up-to-date information about the natural history of the infectious agent, demands on the system, and resource availability.[1,35]

2. A centralised triage advisory committee with command and control over resources (this may require legislative support).[1,35]

3. An efficient communications network that allows two-way communications between the 'field' (hospitals) and the command centre.

4. Trained triage officers in the field with the authority to make and enforce triage decisions.[35]

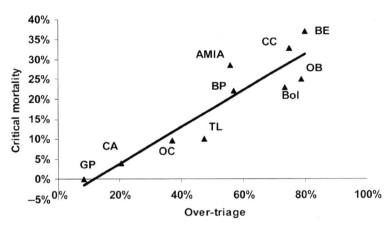

Fig. 10.5 Impact of over-triage on survival. Graphic relation of over-triage rate to critical mortality rate, in 10 terrorist bombing incidents from 1969 to 1995. Linear correlation coefficient (r) 0.92; GP, Guildford pubs; CA, Craigavon; OC, Oklahoma City; TL, Tower of London; BP, Birmingham pubs; Bol, Bologna; AMIA, Buenos Aires; OB, Old Bailey; CC, Cu Chi; BE, Beirut.[35] Source: Frykberg.[35]

efforts should be focused during the preparedness phase is the development of the infrastructure necessary to allow effective triage (Table 10.4).

Accurate triage is critical to maximise survival. Triaging patients inappropriately to critical care is called 'over-triage'.[35] Over-triage results in inappropriate resource expenditures. Frykberg[35] showed that over-triage of patients involved in terrorist bombings is directly related to overall increased mortality rates (Fig. 10.5). Real-time data about patient outcomes during a biological disaster are required to allow modification of the triage criteria in order to prevent under or over-triage. Another possible mechanism to fine tune triage criteria is to use computer modelling based on databases of patients with similar illnesses from non-biological occurrences (e.g. influenza). The utility of such modelling was demonstrated by Garner and his colleagues during their work on trauma triage guidelines.[57]

Infection control

Infection control is a key component of any response involving an infectious bioagent. As was demonstrated during SARS, HCWs and patients in the critical care environment are particularly vulnerable to nosocomial transmission of infectious agents, owing to invasive procedures such as intubation, suctioning, central line insertion, etc.[5,8,10,11,12,13,58] This highlights the need for infection control to be incorporated into all disaster planning.[9] However, infection control should not just be seen as an important issue during crises; ensuring good day-to-day infection control practices and staff education is the best way to prepare for disasters.

The basic approach to infection control in critical care units should consider administrative controls, environmental engineering, protective equipment, and quality control.[5] The primary goal of infection control is to prevent transmission to HCWs and others. Cohorting of patients who are likely or unlikely to be infectious is an important first step in containing the spread of illness and is facilitated through use of the SEIRV protocol.[37] During a biological disaster involving an infectious agent, separate ICUs should be developed to deal with infectious and non-infectious patients. For example a hospital with a single medical–surgical ICU and a coronary care unit (CCU) could designate its medical–surgical ICU as the 'infectious ICU', and then use its post-anaesthetic care unit (PACU) to manage non-infectious surgical patients and the CCU for all non-infectious medical patients requiring critical care. Whilst cohorting should not be relied upon as a foolproof method of infection control, it does significantly decrease the exposure of highly susceptible critically ill patients to potential infection.

Infection control considerations for critical care should begin as early as the design stage of the ICU. Many new ICUs are designed in an open concept with large open spaces using curtains to divide ICU bays as opposed to individual rooms with walls and doors. Such open concepts are aesthetically pleasing but they do not allow for efficient infection control or isolation. New ICUs should be designed to allow isolation of individual patients as well as the entire unit. Additionally, airflow issues and other environmental controls must also be considered when designing and constructing critical care units. Similarly, when planning alternative critical care locations during a surge, infection control issues must also be considered. One option includes the use of portable 'high efficiency particulate filtration' (HEPA) filters to create negative pressure units.[59] Finally, some procedures in the ICU require higher levels of personal protection, given they have the potential to generate aerosols thus increasing the risk of airborne transmission even for infectious agents that would otherwise typically only be transmitted via droplets.[5,8,12,13] Additional precautions and possibly the use of special procedure rooms should be considered for high-risk procedures.

In terms of patient isolation and personal protective equipment, generally four types of precautions are used. The first are 'standard precautions' and they apply to any exposures to blood, body fluids (all secretions and excretions except sweat, regardless of whether or not they contain visible blood), non-intact skin, and mucous membranes regardless of the presumed infectious status of the patient. Hand hygiene should always be used in addition to various personal protective equipment (PPE) such as gloves, gowns, masks, and eye protection as indicated. The other three forms of precautions are implemented based on the presumed infectious status of a patient. These include:

- Contact precautions: gloves, gowns and hand hygiene

- Droplet precautions: a surgical mask and eye protection

- Airborne precautions: N95 mask

Although we have listed the specific PPE used with each type of precaution, three important points must also be remembered:

- These precautions are always applied in addition to standard precautions

- Occasionally precautions are combined, i.e. 'droplet/contact' for specific infections

- Other infection-control measures such as environmental engineering controls also play an important role in these precautions

A full discussion of infection control practices in critical care is beyond the scope of this chapter and interested readers should refer to excellent articles discussing the transmission of respiratory pathogens[60] or bioterrorism agents.[61]

A common theme that has been revisited throughout this chapter is the need for real-time data to guide decision-making and responses. This is also true for infection control as was demonstrated during SARS. In Toronto we learned that during a biological disaster, even more important than the initiation of the response is the transition from response to recovery. Simply put, how to detect and respond to an outbreak was well understood, but how to end an outbreak was not. The failure to detect an ongoing chain of SARS transmission in a hospital led to a second large wave of infections and deaths after infection-control precautions were discontinued.[6,7] Appropriate surveillance data could have detected and prevented this second wave of illness.

Ethical challenges

Given the life-and-death stakes associated with many of the critical care issues it is not surprising that a number of ethical challenges arise. Ethical issues related to resource allocation were discussed earlier. This section will discuss an issue that was brought to the forefront of discussion during SARS: the duty of HCWs to provide care. Severe acute respiratory syndrome SARS was associated with both physical and psychological risks to HCWs.[9,33,62,63] As a result of this, some HCWs refused to work or demanded hazard pay. This reaction was not unique to SARS. Similar issues were faced during the early days of the acquired immunodeficiency syndrome (AIDS) epidemic[64] and will likely be seen with future emerging infectious diseases.[65] It is important that those planning critical care responses to biological disasters consider such issues, given their human resources supply implications as well as the human impact on their HCWs.

Conclusion

Critical care units are likely to be significantly impacted by a biological disaster as well as being particularly vulnerable to nosocomial transmissions. A critical care response to bioterrorism and outbreaks require preparation, training, and a well-organised/controlled response. When patient volumes exceed normal limits surge capacity, mass critical care and triage are invaluable tools required to achieve the goal of saving as many lives as possible. Appropriate infection control techniques are critical to saves lives by preventing secondary transmission to health care workers or other patients.

Acknowledgements

The authors wish to thank Paul Moir for his assistance with the design and production of the graphics within this chapter.

References

1. Rubinson L, O'Toole T. Critical care during epidemics. *Crit Care* 2005; **9**: 311–13.
2. Christian MD, Poutanen SM, Loutfy MR, Muller MP, Low DE. Severe acute respiratory syndrome. *Clin Infect Dis* 2004; **38**: 1420–27.

3. Booth CM, Matukas LM, Tomlinson GA *et al*. Clinical features and short-term outcomes of 144 patients with SARS in the greater Toronto area. *JAMA* 2003; **289**: 2801–09.

4. Poutanen SM, Low DE, Henry B *et al*. Identification of severe acute respiratory syndrome in Canada. *N Engl J Med* 2003; **348**: 1995–2005.

5. Christian MD, Loutfy M, McDonald LC *et al*. Possible SARS coronavirus transmission during cardiopulmonary resuscitation. *Emerg Infect Dis* 2004; **10**: 287–93.

6. Wallington T, Berger L, Henry B *et al*. Update: severe acute respiratory syndrome – Toronto, 2003. *Can Commun Dis Rep* 2003; **29**: 113–17.

7. Wong T, Wallington T, McDonald LC *et al*. Late recognition of SARS in nosocomial outbreak, Toronto. *Emerg Infect Dis* 2005; **11**: 322–5.

8. Fowler RA, Guest CB, Lapinsky SE *et al*. Transmission of severe acute respiratory syndrome during intubation and mechanical ventilation. *Am J Respir Crit Care Med* 2004; **169**: 1198–202.

9. Hawryluck L, Lapinsky S, Stewart T. Clinical review: SARS – lessons in disaster management. *Crit Care* 2005; **9**: 384–9.

10. Lapinsky SE, Hawryluck L. ICU management of severe acute respiratory syndrome. *Intensive Care Med* 2003; **29**: 870–5.

11. Lapinsky SE, Granton JT. Critical care lessons from severe acute respiratory syndrome. *Curr Opin Crit Care* 2004; **10**: 53–8.

12. Ofner M, Lem M, Sarwal S, Vearncombe M, Simor A. Cluster of severe acute respiratory syndrome cases among protected health care workers Toronto, April 2003. *Can Commun Dis Rep* 2003; **29**: 93–7.

13. Scales DC, Green K, Chan AK *et al*. Illness in intensive care staff after brief exposure to severe acute respiratory syndrome. *Emerg Infect Dis* 2003; **9**: 1205–10.

14. Karwa M, Bronzert P, Kvetan V. Bioterrorism and critical care. *Crit Care Clin* 2003; **19**: 279–313.

15. Andresen M. "Imminent" flu pandemic: Are we ready? *CMAJ* 2004; **170**: 181.

16. Fauci AS. Pandemic influenza threat and preparedness. *Emerg Infect Dis* 2006; **12**: 73–7.

17. Osterholm MT. Preparing for the next pandemic. *N Engl J Med* 2005; **352**: 1839–42.

18. Koopmans M, Wilbrink B, Conyn M *et al*. Transmission of H7N7 avian influenza A virus to human beings during a large outbreak in commercial poultry farms in the Netherlands. *Lancet* 2004; **363**: 587–93.

19. Webster RG, Peiris M, Chen H, Guan Y. H5N1 outbreaks and enzootic influenza. *Emerg Infect Dis* 2006; **12**: 3–8.

20. Schoch-Spana M. Implications of pandemic influenza for bioterrorism response. *Clin Infect Dis* 2000; **31**: 1409–13.

21. Christian MD, Kollek D, Schwartz B. Emergency preparedness: what every healthcare worker needs to know. *Can J Emerg Med* 2005; **7**: 330–7.

22. Dara SI, Ashton RW, Farmer JC. Engendering enthusiasm for sustainable disaster critical care response: why is this of consequence to critical care professionals? *Crit Care* 2005; **9**: 125–7.

23. Gani R, Hughes H, Fleming D *et al*. Potential impact of antiviral drug use during influenza pandemic. *Emerg Infect Dis* 2005; **11**: 1355–62.

24. Hirshberg A, Stein M, Walden R. Surgical resource utilization in urban terrorist bombing: a computer simulation. *J Trauma* 1999; **47**: 545–50.

25. Smith DJ. Predictability and preparedness in influenza control. *Science* 2006; **312**: 392–4.
26. Christen H, Maniscalco P, Vickery A, Winslow F. *An Overview of Incident Management Systems*, 4, 2001. Belfer Center for Science and International Affairs, Harvard University: http://bcsia.ksg.harvard.edu/BCSIA_content/documents/An_Overview_of_Incident_Management_Systems.pdf.
27. Shamir MY, Weiss YG, Willner D *et al*. Multiple casualty terror events: the anesthesiologist's perspective. *Anesth Analg* 2004; **98**: 1746–52.
28. Honorable Mr Justice Archie Campbell. *The SARS Commission Interim Report: SARS and Public Health in Ontario* 2004; 12.
29. Naylor D, Basrur S, Bergeron MG *et al*. *A Report of the National Advisory Committee on SARS and Public Health Learning from SARS – Renewal in Public Health in Canada* 2003. http://www.phac-aspc.gc.ca/publicat/sars-sras/naylor/.
30. United States of America Federal Emergency Measures Agency. *National Incident Management. Homeland Security, System* 2004. http://training.fema.gov/EMIWeb/IS/ICS Resource/assets/NIMS-90-web.pdf.
31. Hick JL, Hanfling D, Burstein JL *et al*. Health care facility and community strategies for patient care surge capacity. *Ann Emerg Med* 2004; **44**: 253–61.
32. Cushman JG, Pachter HL, Beaton HL. Two New York City hospitals' surgical response to the September 11, 2001, terrorist attack in New York City. *J Trauma* 2003; **54**: 147–54.
33. Booth CM, Stewart TE. Communication in the Toronto critical care community: important lessons learned during SARS. *Crit Care* 2003; **7**: 405–6.
34. Klein JS, Weigelt JA. Disaster management. Lessons learned. *Surg Clin North Am* 1991; **71**: 257–66.
35. Frykberg ER. Medical management of disasters and mass casualties from terrorist bombings: how can we cope? *J Trauma* 2002; **53**: 201–12.
36. Lim S, Closson T, Howard G, Gardam M. Collateral damage: the unforeseen effects of emergency outbreak policies. *Lancet Infect Dis* 2004; **4**: 697–703.
37. Burkle FM, Jr. Mass casualty management of a large-scale bioterrorist event: an epidemiological approach that shapes triage decisions. *Emerg Med Clin North Am* 2002; **20**: 409–36.
38. Fine MJ, Stone RA, Lave JR *et al*. Implementation of an evidence-based guideline to reduce duration of intravenous antibiotic therapy and length of stay for patients hospitalized with community-acquired pneumonia: a randomized controlled trial. *Am J Med* 2003; **115**: 343–51.
39. Hauck LD, Adler LM, Mulla ZD. Clinical pathway care improves outcomes among patients hospitalized for community-acquired pneumonia. *Ann Epidemiol* 2004; **14**: 669–75.
40. Marrie TJ, Lau CY, Wheeler SL *et al*. A controlled trial of a critical pathway for treatment of community-acquired pneumonia. CAPITAL Study Investigators. Community-Acquired Pneumonia Intervention Trial Assessing Levofloxacin. *JAMA* 2000; **283**: 749–55.
41. Ontario Ministry of Health and Long Term Care. *Ontario Health Pandemic Influenza Plan*. 2006. http://www.health.gov.on.ca/english/providers/program/emu/pan_flu/pan_flu_plan.html.

42. Public Health Agency of Canada. *Canadian Pandemic Influenza Plan*. 2005. http://www.phac-aspc.gc.ca/cpip-pclcpi/index.html.
43. University of Toronto Joint Centre for Bioethics Pandemic Influenza Working Group. *Stand On Guard For Thee: Ethical Considerations in Preparedness Planning for Pandemic Influenza*. 2005. http://www.utoronto.ca/jcb/home/documents/pandemic.pdf.
44. Domres B, Koch M, Manger A, Becker HD. Ethics and triage. *Prehospital Disaster Med* 2001; **16**: 53–8.
45. Baskett PJ. Ethics in disaster medicine. *Prehospital Disaster Med* 1994; **9**: 4–5.
46. Vollmar LC. Military medicine in war: the Geneva Conventions today. In: Thomas E. Beam, Linette R.Sparacino, eds., *Military Medical Ethics*. Washington, DC: Office of The Surgeon General Department of the Army, United States of America, 2003.
47. Murray M, Bullard M, Grafstein E. Revisions to the Canadian Emergency Department Triage and Acuity Scale Implementation Guidelines. *Can J Emerg Med* 2004; **6**: 421–7.
48. Ethical issues. Health Disaster Management: Guidelines for Evaluation and Research in the "Utstein Style". *Prehospital Disaster Med* 17 2002; **17** (Suppl 3): 128–43.
49. Knaus WA, Zimmerman JE, Wagner DP, Draper EA, Lawrence DE. APACHE-acute physiology and chronic health evaluation: a physiologically based classification system. *Crit Care Med* 1981; **9**: 591–7.
50. Knaus WA, Draper EA, Wagner DP, Zimmerman JE. APACHE II: a severity of disease classification system. *Crit Care Med* 1985; **13**: 818–29.
51. Knaus WA, Wagner DP, Draper EA *et al*. The APACHE III prognostic system. Risk prediction of hospital mortality for critically ill hospitalized adults. *Chest* 1991; **100**: 1619–36.
52. Christian MD, Hawryluck L, Wax RS *et al*. A triage protocol for critical care during a pandemic. *CMAJ* 2006; **175**: 1377–81.
53. Ferreira FL, Bota DP, Bross A, Melot C, Vincent JL. Serial evaluation of the SOFA score to predict outcome in critically ill patients. *JAMA* 2001; **286**: 1754–58.
54. Benson M, Koenig KL, Schultz CH. Disaster triage: START, then SAVE – a new method of dynamic triage for victims of a catastrophic earthquake. *Prehospital Disaster Med* 1996; **11**: 117–24.
55. Risavi BL, Salen PN, Heller MB, Arcona S. A two-hour intervention using START improves prehospital triage of mass casualty incidents. *Prehosp Emerg Care* 2001; **5**: 197–9.
56. Romig LE. Pediatric triage. A system to jump start your triage of young patients at MCIs. *JEMS* 2002; **27**: 52–3.
57. Garner A, Lee A, Harrison K, Schultz CH. Comparative analysis of multiple-casualty incident triage algorithms. *Ann Emerg Med* 2001; **38**: 541–8.
58. Fowler RA, Lapinsky SE, Hallett D *et al*. Critically ill patients with severe acute respiratory syndrome. *JAMA* 2003; **290**: 367–73.
59. Rosenbaum RA, Benyo JS, O'Connor RE *et al*. Use of a portable forced air system to convert existing hospital space into a mass casualty isolation area. *Ann Emerg Med* 2004; **44**: 628–34.
60. Muller MP, McGeer A. Febrile respiratory illness in the intensive care unit setting: an infection control perspective. *Curr Opin Crit Care* 2006; **12**: 37–42.

61. Karwa M, Currie B, Kvetan V. Bioterrorism: preparing for the impossible or the improbable. *Crit Care Med* 2005; **33**(Suppl 1): S75–S95.
62. Gold W, Hawryluck L, Robinson S, McGreer A, Styra R. *Post-traumatic Stress Disorder (PTSD) among Healthcare Workers (HCW) at a Hospital Treating Patients with SARS* (abstract). Chicago, IL: presented at 43rd Interscience Conference on Antimicrobial Agents and Chemotherapy (ICAAC); 14–17 September 2003; K–750a.
63. Straus SE, Wilson K, Rambaldini G *et al.* Severe acute respiratory syndrome and its impact on professionalism: qualitative study of physicians' behaviour during an emerging healthcare crisis. *BMJ* 2004; **329**: 83.
64. Loewy EH. Duties, fears and physicians. *Soc Sci Med* 1986; **22**: 1363–6.
65. Alexander GC, Wynia MK. Ready and willing? Physicians' sense of preparedness for bioterrorism. *Health Aff (Millwood)* 2003; **22**: 189–97.

Hannah Barrett, Alison D. Bullock and Julian F. Bion

Evaluating clinical performance

Making judgements about ourselves and others is a universal human phenomenon repeated daily in social intercourse, examination halls, or courts of law. It is the desire to do this in an objective, repeatable, reliable and constructive manner that underpins the principle of professional self-regulation. However, this principle has been challenged by evidence of error in healthcare worldwide,[1,2,3,4,5,6,7] and in the UK by several high-profile individual failures which have exposed flaws in regulatory systems. The subsequent public enquiries and their reports[8,9,10,11] have stimulated modifications to training and assessment including regular appraisal and continuing professional development to ensure competence,[8] introduction of a national system for reviewing doctors in difficulty,[12] and several reviews of the concept of professionalism.[13,14,15,16] In short, we will only retain the high level of public trust currently accorded to the medical profession if we combine effective assessment of competence with continued monitoring of performance.[17,18] Assessment is thus an essential part of ensuring safe and effective patient care.

So much is obvious. But are we not doing this already? The medical profession has from earliest times made a commitment to place the interests of the patient before those of the practitioner and to maintain the highest standards of practice through examination and peer review. The problem is that this commitment may not be shared by all members of the profession. The absence of explicit standards and transparency makes assessment of performance difficult and therefore limits accountability. In addition the systems of self-regulation and professional development designed in the nineteenth century are insufficient instruments for the complexities of modern healthcare.

Recent Advances in Anaesthesia and Intensive Care 24, ed. J. N. Cashman and R. M. Grounds.
Published by Cambridge University Press. © Cambridge University Press 2007.

Until relatively recently, assessment and maintenance of quality of medical practice relied on a system of hurdles or barriers, the two most prominent being the transition from undergraduate to qualified hospital general practitioner ('generalist') and from generalist to specialist. Once these barriers were passed, all that was required was regular clinical practice and the confidence of one's patients and colleagues. This system lacked certain key elements: it was summative (final assessment) as opposed to formative (educational, developmental), it focused more on knowledge and less on skills and attitudes, and there was no continued monitoring function to detect and correct sub-optimal practice and protect patients. A modern system of regulation and professional development requires all these elements.

Approaches vary worldwide in terms of the extent to which education (professional development) and regulation (revalidation, recertification) are linked, the methods used, and their legal force.[19] Regular recertification is now routine in the United States of America, Canada, Australia and New Zealand. In the USA, where regular recertification is the norm, methods vary between Speciality Boards, but often include a multiple choice examination,[20] with formal approval of educational materials by the Accreditation Council for Continuing Medical Education. Canada and Australia have voluntary systems of continuing medical education, whilst New Zealand mandates participation in formal professional development programmes for recertification. Europe, however, has been slow to follow, with the majority of countries having voluntary systems of education credits (generally one point per hour of activity). Only the Netherlands has a mandatory system of recertification.

In the UK this is set to change with the report by Sir Liam Donaldson, the Chief Medical Officer for England, '*Good Doctors, Safer Patients*'.[21] This seminal publication makes 44 recommendations about the regulation and professional development of doctors. The likely outcome will be a mandated system which links appraisal, professional development and recertification. Donaldson calls, *inter alia*, for 'a greater emphasis on retraining and rehabilitation...regular assessment of standards [and] strengthening and standardising the system of annual appraisal'.

Defining performance

In recent years national regulatory bodies for doctors have started to modify their training programmes from syllabus-based examination-driven systems to those based on competencies which define the outcomes of training in terms of knowledge, skills, attitudes and behaviours, assessed in the workplace. This important shift focuses attention on what doctors should be able to do (viz. their clinical performance), and on the needs of

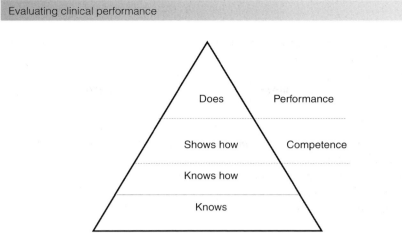

Fig. 11.1a The assessment of clinical skills and competence/performance according to Miller.[22]

the patients they serve, rather than solely assessing what they know. It also permits identification of common elements between disciplines which, in theory at least, should enhance multidisciplinary teamworking and provides a useful reference point for maintenance of specialist competence.

Miller's hierarchy of learning illustrates that assessment targets for undergraduate training have greater focus on the acquisition of knowledge and less on performance in practice (Figure 11.1a).[22] In contrast, postgraduate training places an increasing importance on performance and assessment strategies and must therefore focus at the 'action' or 'does' level.[23] The Cambridge model incorporates this concept by inverting Miller's triangle and brings additional components in the form of systems (context and environment) factors and individual (personal) factors (Figure 11.1b).[24]

Definitions of competencies serve to guide the assessment processes. Descriptions of what doctors should be able to do create a benchmark against which judgements can be made of clinical performance. Without such definitions, judgements of clinical performance are open to varied interpretations of what it is to be a 'good' doctor. However, competence-based systems are not without their critics. Criticisms of competence-based training include the view that it sets a minimum standard instead of aspiring to excellence, that it reduces professionals to the level of craftsmen, that the complexity of 'being a good doctor' cannot be reduced to a simple list of tasks or activities and that it fails to acknowledge the context and evolution of professional competence.[25,26,27]

A commonly expressed concern is 'how do I know that this trainee is competent?'. The trainee journeys towards safe, independent practice, achieving

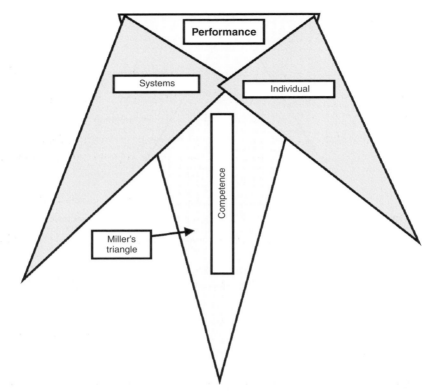

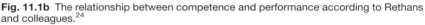

Fig. 11.1b The relationship between competence and performance according to Rethans and colleagues.[24]

competencies along the way. A summative judgement of safe, independent practice is based on an accumulation of assessments. But clinical performance is a changing quantity (competencies gained or lost) and needs to be regularly reviewed. To do this requires reliable methods of work-place based assessments which allow us to make judgements about a clinician's abilities (performance).

Evaluating performance

Features of good assessment

In the UK, the Postgraduate Medical Education and Training Board (PMETB) is charged with setting appropriate standards for assessments. The PMETB has published guidance, albeit in draft form, on the assessment framework required.[28] In principle three it states: 'Methods will be chosen on the basis of validity, reliability, feasibility, cost-effectiveness, opportunities for feedback, and impact on learning.' These concepts are considered in turn.

Validity and reliability
Different forms of validity include:

- Face validity. Does the assessment measure what it purports to measure?

- Content validity. To what degree does the assessment represent the content that the test is designed to measure?

- Concurrent validity. Does performance on the assessment tasks match that obtained in other assessments of the same group of trainees taken at roughly the same time?

- Intrinsic validity. Do the assessment tasks measure the learning objectives of the course?

- Extrinsic validity. Are the objectives of the programme desirable/good in themselves?

- Predictive validity. Do the assessment tasks predict future performance accurately?

Ensuring that assessments are valid can be challenging and, too often, claims of validity lack clarity.

Reliable assessment is objective, accurate, repeatable and analytically sound. An objective assessment is one that is not compromised by observer bias. This is unproblematic when the focus is on what can be objectively measured, but a challenge for much workplace-based observation where there is a need to assess complex performance that may be ill-defined. The more we simplify, the more reliable the assessment. However, such simplification fails to reflect the complexity of human behaviour. For complex skills like clinical competence this is not easy. In addition agreed definitions of what counts as good evidence are needed. Nevertheless reliability can be enhanced by assessor training, monitoring and second and third observers. This is costly. In terms of accuracy, the measurement must be stable (objective, repeatable and consistent between observers over time) and sensitive (able to detect important variations in performance). An analytically sound assessment is one correctly marked, using agreed grading criteria. Numerical data from different sources should not be merged otherwise the meaning of the resulting number is lost.

Validity and reliability may conflict in complex tasks. One might ask which matters most? For learning outcomes that can be readily determined (for example, knowledge-based tests relying on information recall) then reliability is perhaps more important. For complex learning outcomes, putting reliability first may result in tests that simplify complexity and provide information about something quite different from that intended.

Some would argue that all assessment is subjective. The task is to make judgments defensible and credible. However, Guba and Lincoln have suggested alternative criteria: credibility, transferability and dependability.[29] Credibility parallels internal validity (how the assessment relates to the learning objectives) and involves establishing a match between the assessment and the fuzzy realities of those being assessed, the assessors and other stakeholders. Assessment methodologies which allow work to be viewed over a period of time (rather than one-off exams) are favoured. Transferability relates to external validity or generalisability and is concerned with the extent to which findings from assessments are transferable. Here 'thick description', including a careful description of the time, place, context and the culture relative to the assessment, is important. Dependability parallels reliability. Here it is recognised that it is normal and desirable that assessment views change. Dependability is encouraged by an open process whereby assessment views are challenged and open to criticism.

Feasibility and cost-effectiveness
Good assessments are also those which can be undertaken within the constraints of time, staff and finances. Assessments should fit well with the training programme and the working day. If these more practical considerations are overlooked, even the slickest assessment procedure will fail to be implemented.

Feedback and learning
Assessment should provide good feedback and encourage learning; assessment procedures should help the trainee identify strengths and weaknesses. There are strong positive links between assessment, good feedback and further learning. The purpose of formative assessment is to provide feedback on progress and encourage learning. Assessment is an educational and diagnostic activity, concerned with the identification of strengths and weaknesses, the demonstration of achievement (triangulated across a range of assessments) and the signalling of where more practice or support is needed.

Regarding the identification of weakness, a good assessment system will detect poor performance early in the training programme. Poor clinical performance may become manifest in different ways. For the trainee it may be rooted in either adaptive or personal causes. In general the adaptive causes are more difficult to manage and are most often seen as:

- Failure to integrate knowledge into clinical practice. This is often seen as inappropriate ranking of differential diagnoses and poor choice of diagnostic tests.

- Attitudes which are overly hierarchical, intolerant of advice and demonstrate poor leadership skills. These may stem from poor role models or a rigid personality.

Personal causes have many origins including:

- Illness; commonly psychological, but sometimes physical.

- Indulgence; excessive use of alcohol, drugs and too active a social life.

- Internal conflicts owing to cultural dislocation or religious incompatibility with medical practice.

- Difficulties in interpersonal relationships.

It would be naïve to suggest that each of these problems occurs in isolation or just in trainees. A feature of a good assessment procedure is one that can identify poor performance early on so that remedial action may be taken (although not all problems are remediable).

Tools for assessment

There are a range of methods and tools in use to assess training but assessment of doctors' performance at work is in its infancy.[30] The content and difficulty of the 'test' cannot be controlled in this context. Instead assessment must be based on the responses of the doctor to the patients that he/she encounters. Assessment must go beyond technical skills to include the doctor's communication skills, whether or not the doctor is up to date, whether or not the doctor involves patients in treatment decisions and whether or not the doctor affords their patients dignity and respect. Central to the evaluation of clinical performance is assessment in the workplace.

Workplace-based assessment methods

Workplace-based assessments have primarily been developed for use during medical training but they are wholly relevant to any evaluation of performance. The closer the assessment is to the performance under scrutiny, the more it is authentic. Performance ('does') can only be demonstrated under real conditions, in the real workplace environment. Performance can only be implied from assessments of 'shows how' (for example in a simulation exercise). Such exercises are not without worth in the evaluation of clinical performance. However, they are necessarily secondary to workplace-based assessments, the most important of which is observation.

Observation   This is the most commonly used approach to competence assessment and may be described as the traditional 'apprentice–master' model of training. It requires frequent observation by an experienced trainer and works well for the majority of trainees. Interactions during routine clinical work offer frequent opportunities for informal observation by different members of the healthcare team and on a number of occasions. Over a period of time these encounters provide a general overview of the doctor's performance to allow feedback of strengths or weaknesses, identify future learning needs, or indicate the need for further assessment based on direct observation using specific tools if problems are identified.

Observations may be formally structured and documented by using a variety of assessment tools, selected according to whether specific knowledge, skills and/or behavioural aspects of practice are being assessed. Examples include:

- Direct observation of procedural skills (DOPS). Direct observation of a doctor performing diagnostic and interventional procedures during normal ('routine') clinical practice is used to assess the doctor–patient interaction and the process as a whole, not just the procedure itself. The assessment is recorded using a structured check-list which enables the assessor to provide feedback.[31,32]

- Clinical evaluation exercise (CEX). A 'snapshot' observation of a normal ('routine') clinical encounter for a limited period of time (e.g. five minutes) or for the complete period of the patient encounter according to the assessment tool in use. Designed to assess clinical skills, attitudes and behaviours.[33,34]

- Multi-source feedback (MSF). MSF (also termed 360° assessment, peer assessment or team assessment of behaviour), seeks the views of members of the healthcare team on the doctor's professional attitudes and behaviour in day-to-day work. Forms are distributed by the doctor to a predetermined number of raters; completed forms are returned to a central point and are summarised. Feedback is then provided during a meeting between the doctor and the reviewer. The numbers of raters and the format of the rating scale vary according to the tool in use.[35,36,37,38]

- Anaesthetists' non-technical skills behavioural marker system (ANTS). In the area of anaesthetists' non-technical skills (task and resource management, team working, situation awareness and decision-making) a behavioural marker system has been developed which identifies good and poor behaviour and allows feedback to be given to doctors about the non-technical aspects of their performance.[39] Although further work is required to develop protocols and training programmes for the users of the system, an evaluation study has demonstrated that it is a valid, reliable and practical tool for observing and rating behaviour in real-time training situations (see Chapter 12).[40]

Case reviews and analysis   Although not based on direct observation of performance, review or analysis of cases is a good indicator of performance.

- Structured case histories. These are used both as a learning and assessment opportunity. A written report summarises a case that has been encountered and, with reference to relevant literature, reflects upon the management of this case. A minimum number of case summaries (the UK intensive care programme requires ten)[41] are completed during training and submitted to the educational supervisor/trainer who confirms that they have been completed to an acceptable standard. The topic is selected by the trainee in discussion with the trainer, with the aim of covering a broad range of topics relevant to clinical practice in order to complement an area of special interest, provide evidence of competence related to prior experience or help to improve an area of weakness for the trainee.

- Case-based discussion. Used to explore clinical reasoning and management. The patient record of a challenging clinical case is the focus of a structured discussion between the doctor and reviewer.[41,42,43,44] Termed 'Chart Stimulated Recall' in North America,[44] it allows the doctor to explain the reasoning behind choices they have made and provides an opportunity for the discussion of the ethical and legal framework of practice. An assessment form is completed by the reviewer who then provides immediate feedback to the doctor in order to guide learning.

- Analysis of clinical processes and outcomes. It has been suggested that judgements may be made on the basis of processes of care, patient outcomes, and volume, taking into account threats to validity and reliability such as case mix and complexity.[30] As electronic systems of data-capture and decision-support become more widespread, we should evaluate their utility as measures of medical performance. This might include adherence to best-practice guidelines when a patient is first admitted, procedure-related complications such as bacteraemia rates associated with central venous catheter placement, or complaints or compliments from patients or relatives. Process measures are more useful measures of performance whilst mortality rates are unlikely to be reliable measures because of confounding factors.

Assessments outside the workplace

Simulations (including OSCEs).   Simulations (artificial representation of real situations) allow skills to be practised in a safe and controlled environment. They can also be used for assessment of decision-making, communication and technical skills.[45,46] A simulation may use mannequins, 'standardised patients' or computer-based programmes according to the purpose of the assessment, which may be much like workplace-based observation. They may be part of an OSCE (objective structured clinical examination), standardised clinical problems presented at a number of stations in a simulation centre, or skills laboratory. However, simulations are resource-, cost- and time-intensive. They cannot take the place of direct experience with real patients.

Formal knowledge-based examination.   Formal examination is of course the method most widely used to make judgements about a doctor's ability. Formal knowledge tests, for example using multiple choice examinations, are easy to apply and have the attraction of numerical end points which may demonstrate a relationship with certain aspects of clinician behaviour or quality of practice.[47] However, few would argue that knowledge-based examinations are necessarily good indicators of practical competence in the clinical environment. They are best used to ensure a certain standard of knowledge acquisition, and can be seen as quality indicators to supplement the 'safe practitioner' approach of workplace-based assessment of competence. Formal knowledge-based examination and workplace-based assessment of competence are complementary.

Assessment and appraisal

These two processes are complementary but serve different purposes.

Assessment

Assessment concerns external measurements and judgements of clinical or other relevant professional competence or performance. Assessments are used to judge the effectiveness of periods of training, to measure the readiness of a trainee to proceed to further periods of employment or training, and to provide safeguards of minimum standards of patient care. A good assessment procedure will encourage learning through the provision of feedback. In all the assessments described here, feedback is a central component of the process.[48] The purpose of this type of formative assessment is to shed light on areas of strength and weakness. The data from these assessments inform the trainee's learning requirements, or what the experienced doctor needs to do to sustain or enhance performance. Such reflection on learning needs should shape the choice of continuing professional development activity. Feedback on assessment will usually take place at an appraisal meeting.

Appraisal

Appraisal uses self-examination and reflection to encourage both the individual practitioner and the (employing) organisation to move current practice towards some notion of desired practice. This results in either confirmation of practice (assurance) or identification of educational needs accompanied by actions to address shortcomings. The value of this type of formative assessment in facilitating learning is clear. Such formative assessment can help learners reflect and transform their experience.

Logbooks and portfolios

These are important sources of evidence to facilitate both assessment and appraisal. A logbook is a record which provides evidence of experience. It is used to record patients treated (identifying practical skills and procedures), training placements, teaching programmes undertaken, courses or conferences attended, audits, publications etc. It informs educational agreements and may assist in the trainee's reflections on progress and learning. Though logbooks may play a part in assessment, they are not in themselves a form of assessment, nor does the completion of a logbook provide any inherent guarantee of quality of training or experience unless it is associated with a measure of the quality of the work completed.

Maintaining performance

Undergraduates

There is no common curriculum for training in resuscitation and acute care at undergraduate level, although in the UK the GMC expects all doctors to be able to offer care in an emergency.[49] The Acute Care Undergraduate Teaching initiative[50] has used consensus techniques to develop a curriculum in resuscitation and acute care for undergraduates, and this will integrate well with generic (Foundation Years) training in acute care for junior doctors in the UK.[51] The model is transferable to other countries. These developments will provide a continuum with postgraduate critical care training programmes. The challenge lies in resourcing and valuing training and methods of assessment. Universities often pay lip service to the importance of education, whilst continuing to judge academic staff predominantly on their research output. More attention should be paid to the quality of teaching and training, since it is at this early stage in career development that dysfunctional attitudes and behaviours may become set, emerging later in life as professional failure or patient harm.[52]

Doctors in training grades

In contrast to undergraduate training where the focus is more on the acquisition of knowledge, postgraduate training places increasing importance on performance. Assessment strategies must therefore focus at the 'action' or 'does' level.[23] Apart from the major issue of standardisation of assessment of competence and selection of appropriate methods, which have been discussed above, the challenge for trainers as busy clinicians is to find sufficient time and frequent enough opportunities to undertake the assessments of trainees' competence during routine work. This is a particular issue in an environment where there are numerous trainees working shifts, as they may only be exposed to individual trainers infrequently. Whilst one specialist will therefore usually be assigned the task of co-ordinating the training programme, it should be the responsibility of all specialists to contribute to the process of teaching and assessment and to find opportunities to discuss individual trainees together in order to develop a degree of commonality in standards of assessment. Assessments of professionalism (predominantly attitudes and behaviour) may, indeed should, also be made by nursing staff and others who are closely acquainted with the individual practitioners (multisource feedback). The transparency of the whole assessment process is substantially improved by the use of educational agreements or personal learning plans.[53] These formalise what the trainee agrees to achieve, and what the training environment guarantees to deliver. They are valuable adjuncts to competency assessment, particularly when evaluating and supporting a trainee in difficulty.

Specialists

In the UK each year around 1% of specialists will develop problems requiring some form of assessment and intervention.[54,55] Data from the UK National Clinical Assessment Service (NCAS) indicate that the reasons for referral to this service include predominantly behavioural problems for younger practitioners, whereas for older practitioners the concerns relate mainly to clinical performance. Referrals increase with age, particularly for family practitioners rather than hospital specialists,[55] whilst clinical capability declines with age.[56] Common sense and experience from high-performance industries such as aviation indicate that the working environment and the degree of mutual support and supervision will determine the extent to which human factors become translated into problems of clinical practice. This has important implications for the continuing monitoring of competence of specialists in terms not only of the methods of assessment, but also the need to assess the professional working environment as much as the practitioner. Consequently, based on work in Canada[57] NCAS assesses performance in four domains: clinical capability, health and well-being, behaviour, and the work environment.

A modern system of regulation and professional development must be able to detect and correct sub-optimal practice and protect patients. It therefore requires a combination of explicit standards combined with process-based, formative assessment focused on knowledge, skills and attitudes, with some elements of summative and outcomes-based assessments.[58,59,60,61] This will require an assessment 'toolbox' containing different measures which can be applied over time by different assessors to common standards. Annual appraisal will include personal portfolios containing evidence of educational activities, and could be combined with measures of group performance to provide a global assessment of institutional quality.

Conclusions

If we are to retain continued public trust in the medical profession we need to take the initiative in effective and transparent professional self-regulation, using predominantly external and objective measures of assessment.[62] The experience of practitioners in countries which have witnessed high-profile failures in duty of care to patients should be an important stimulus for worldwide harmonisation of standards for the acquisition, development and maintenance of professional competence. We need to invest significantly in continuing professional development and in incorporating methods of assessment of competence into routine practice. Recently consensus techniques have been used to develop a comprehensive international competency-based training programme for intensive care medicine – CoBaTrICE – which provides specific guidance on assessment and provides educational resources to assist trainers and trainees.[63] Finally, with the move towards team-based rather than individual-practitioner based care, the organisational environment is an essential element in quality assurance and an area requiring active research and investment by healthcare systems.

References

1. Kohn LT, Corrigan JM, Donaldson MS, eds. *To Err is Human: Building a Safer Health System*. Washington, D.C.: National Academy Press, 2000.
2. Wilson RM, Runciman WB, Gibberd RW, *et al*. The Quality in Australian Health Care Study. *Med J Aust* 1995; **163**: 458–71.

3. Vincent C, Neale G, Woloshynowych M. Adverse events in British hospitals: preliminary retrospective record review. *BMJ* 2001; **322**: 517–19.

4. National Audit Office 2000: www.nao.gov.uk/publications/nao_reports/9900230.

5. Department of Health. *An Organisation with a Memory*. London: Department of Health, 2000. http://www.doh.gov.uk/orgmemreport.

6. Baker GR, Norton P. *Patient Safety and Healthcare Error in the Canadian Healthcare System: A Systematic Review and Analysis of Leading Practices in Canada with Reference to Key Initiatives Elsewhere. A Report to Health Canada*. http://www.hc-sc.gc.ca/english/care/report/index.html.

7. Blendon RJ, DesRoches CM, Brodie M, *et al*. Views of practicing physicians and the public on medical errors. *N Engl J Med* 2002; **347**: 1933–40.

8. The Bristol Royal Infirmary Enquiry. London: Department of Health 2001. http://www.bristol-Inquiry.org.uk/final_report/index.htm.

9. The Department of Health's response to the report of the public inquiry into children's heart surgery at the Bristol Royal Infirmary 1984–1995. http://www.doh.gov.uk/assetRoot/04/05/94/79/04059479.pdf.

10. The Royal Liverpool Children's Enquiry Report 2001. http://www.rlcinquiry.org.uk/download/index.htm.

11. The Shipman Enquiry. http://www.the-shipman-inquiry.org.uk/reports.asp.

12. National Clinical Assessment Service: http://www.ncas.npsa.nhs.uk/.

13. Royal College of Physicians. *Doctors in Society: Medical Professionalism in a Changing World*. Report of a Working Party of the Royal College of Physicians of London. London: Royal College of Physicians, 2005.

14. ABIM Foundation, ACP-ASIM Foundation, European Federation of Internal Medicine. Medical professionalism in the new millennium: a physician's charter. *Ann Intern Med* 2002; **136**: 243–6.

15. Chisholm A, Askham J. *A Review of Professional Codes and Standards For Doctors In the UK, USA, and Canada*. Oxford: Picker Institute Europe, 2006.

16. Hafferty F. Measuring professionalism: a commentary. In: Stern DT, ed., *Measuring Medical Professionalism*. Oxford: Oxford University Press, 2006.

17. http://www.mori.com/polls/2005/bma.shtml.

18. Calnan MW, Sanford E. Public trust in health care: the system or the doctor? *Qual Saf Health Care* 2004; **13**: 92–7.

19. Peck C, McCall M, McLaren B, Rotem T. Continuing medical education and continuing professional development: international comparisons. *BMJ* 2000; **320**: 432–5.

20. Brennan T A. Recertification for internists – one "Grandfather's" experience. *N Engl J Med* 2005; **353**: 1989–2.

21. Chief Medical Officer. *Good Doctors, Safer patients. Proposals to Strengthen the System to Assure and Improve the Performance of Doctors and to Protect the Safety of Patients*. A report by the Chief Medical Officer. London: Department of Health, 2006.

22. Milller GE. The assessment of clinical skills and competence/performance. *Acad Med* 1990; **65**: 563–7.

23. Ringsted C, Skaarup AM, Henriksen AH, Davis D. Person–task-context: a model for designing curriculum and in-training assessment in postgraduate education. *Med Teach* 2006; **28**: 70–6.

24. Rethans JJ, Norcini J, Baron-Maldonado M, *et al*. The relationship between competence and performance: implications for assessing practice performance. *Med Educ* 2002; **36**: 901–9.
25. Harden RM, Crosby JR, Davis MH. AMEE Guide 14: outcome-based education. Part 1 – An introduction to outcome-based education. *Med Teach* 1999; **21**: 7–14.
26. Leung W. Competency-based medical training: review. *BMJ* 2002; **325**: 693–5.
27. Gonczi A. Review of international trends and developments in competency-based education and training. In Argülles A, Gonczi A (eds.), *Competency-Based Education and Training: A World Perspective*. Balderas, Mexico: Noriega Editores; 2000, pp. 15–40.
28. http://www.pmetb.org.uk/media/pdf/1/a/PMETB_quality_assurance_quality_control_and_assessment_systems_guidance_(1_August_2005).pdf.
29. Guba EG, Lincoln YS. *Fourth Generation Evaluation*. London: Sage; 1989.
30. Norcini JJ. Current perspectives in assessment: the assessment of performance at work. *Med Educ* 2005; **39**: 880–9.
31. http://www.mmc.nhs.uk/pages/assessment/dops.
32. http://www.hcat.nhs.uk/foundation/DOPS.htm.
33. http://www.mmc.nhs.uk/pages/assessment/minicex.
34. Norcini JJ, Blank LL, Duffy FD, Fortna GS. The miniCEX: a method for assessing clinical skills. *Ann Int Med* 2003; **138**: 476–81.
35. TAB http://www.mmc.nhs.uk/download_files/360-Team-Assessment-Behaviour-TAB-Form.doc.
36. Mini-PAT http://www.hcat.nhs.uk/foundation/mini-PAT.htm.
37. Ramsey PG, Wenrich MD, Carline JD, Larson EB. Use of peer ratings to evaluate physician performance. *JAMA* 1993; **269**: 1655–60.
38. Evans R, Elwyn G, Edwards A. Review of instruments for peer assessment of physicians. *BMJ* 2004; **328**: 1240.
39. Fletcher G, Flin R, McGeorge P, *et al. The Identification and Measurement of Anaesthetists' Non-Technical Skills: Development of a Prototype Behavioural Marker System for Anaesthetists' Non-Technical Skills (ANTS)* 2003. Industrial Psychology Group, Department of Psychology, University of Aberdeen.
40. Fletcher G, Flin R, McGeorge P, *et al. Evaluation of the Prototype Anaesthetists Non-Technical Skills (ANTS) Behavioural Marker System Experimental Report* 2002. Industrial Psychology Group, Department of Psychology, University of Aberdeen.
41. IBTICM. *The CCST in Intensive Care Medicine: Competency-Based Training and Assessment: Part II (version 6)*. http://www.rcoa.ac.uk/ibticm/docs/CBTPart2.pdf.
42. http://www.mmc.nhs.uk/pages/assessment/cbd.
43. http://www.hcat.nhs.uk/foundation/CbD.htm.
44. ACGME Outcome project (2000). *Toolbox of Assessment Methods*. http://www.acgme.org/Outcome/assess/Toolbox.pdf.
45. Bryne AJ, Greaves JD. Assessment instruments used during anaesthetic simulation: review of published studies. *Br J Anaesth* 2001; **86**: 445–50.
46. Devitt JH, Kurrek MM, Cohen MM, Cleave-Hogg D. The validity of performance assessments using simulation. *Anesthesiology* 2001; **95**: 36–42.
47. Tamblyn R, Abrahamowicz M, Brailovsky C, *et al*. Association between licensing examination scores and resource use and quality of care in primary care practice. *JAMA* 1998; **280**: 989–96.

48. Rushton A. Formative assessment: a key to deep learning? *Med Teach* 2005;
    27: 509–13.
49. General Medical Council, 2001. *Good Medical Practice*. http://www.gmc-uk.
    org/guidance/good_medical_practice/index.asp.
50. Perkins GD, Barrett H, Bullock I, *et al*. The Acute Care Undergraduate
    TEaching (ACUTE) Initiative: consensus development of core competencies in
    acute care for undergraduates in the United Kingdom. *Intensive Care Med*
    2005; **31**: 1627–33.
51. http://www.mmc.nhs.uk/download_files/Curriculum-for-the-foundation-
    years-in-postgraduate-education-and-training.pdf.
52. Papadakis MA, Teherani A, Banach MA, *et al*. Disciplinary action by medical
    boards and prior behavior in medical school. *New Engl J Med* 2005; **353**:
    2673–82.
53. http://www.medev.ac.uk/resources/features/AMEE_summaries/
    AMEE19.pdf.
54. Donaldson L. Doctors with problems in an NHS workforce. *BMJ* 1994; **308**:
    1277–82.
55. National Clinical Assessment Service. *Analysis of the First Four Years'
    Referral Data*. London: National Patient Safety Agency, 2006
    (www.ncas.npsa.nhs.uk).
56. Choudhry N, Fletcher RH, Soumerai SB. Systematic review: the relationship
    between clinical experience and quality of healthcare. *Ann Intern Med* 2005;
    142: 260–73.
57. Dauphinee D. Revalidation of doctors in Canada. *BMJ* 1999; **319**: 1188–90.
58. General Medical Council. *Revalidating Doctors: Ensuring Standards, Securing
    the Future*. London: GMC, 2000.
59. General Medical Council. *A Licence To Practise and Revalidation*. London:
    GMC, 2003.
60. Department of Health. *The Regulation of Non-medical Healthcare
    Professions: A Review by the Department of Health*. London: Department of
    Health, 2006. http://www.dh.gov.uk/assetRoot/04/13/72/95/04137295.pdf.
61. http://www.gmc-uk.org/education/pro_development/pro_development_
    guidance.asp.
62. Davis DA, Mazmanian PE, Fordis M, *et al*. Accuracy of physician self-
    assessment compared with observed measures of competence *JAMA* 2006;
    296: 1094–1102.
63. The CoBaTrICE Collaboration. Consensus development of an international
    competency-based training programme in intensive care medicine. *Intensive
    Care Med* 2006; **32**: 1371–83. www.cobatrice.org.

Other resources and further reading

- Department of Health Appraisal for Doctors in Training: www.dh.
  gov.uk/assetRoot/04/08/03/31/04080331.doc and www.dh.gov.uk/
  assetRoot/04/08/03/27/04080327.doc.

- Department of Health Appraisal for Consultants: www.dh.gov.uk/
  assetRoot/04/03/46/24/04034624.doc.

- Cowan G (ed.). *Assessment and Appraisal of Doctors in Training: Principles and Practice*. Royal College of Physicians (London) 2001.

- Shumway RM, Harden RM. AMEE Guide No. 25: the assessment of learning outcomes for the competent and reflective physician. *Med Teacher* 2003; **25**: 569–84.

- Jolly B, Peyton B. Evaluation. In Peyton JWR, ed., *Teaching and Learning in Medical Practice*. Rickmansworth, UK: Manticore Europe Limited, 1998: pp. 107–15.

- Morrison J. ABC of teaching and learning in medicine: evaluation. *BMJ* 2003; **326**: 385–7, and other articles in this series.

Rona Patey

CHAPTER 12

Non-technical skills and anaesthesia

In 2000 the UK Department of Health published a report entitled '*An Organisation with a Memory*'.[1] This report defined an adverse health care event as 'an event or omission arising during clinical care and causing physical or psychological injury to a patient', and a healthcare near miss as a situation where the events/omissions or sequences of these don't develop further (owing to compensating action or good fortune). Like the earlier US Institute of Medicine report 'To Err is Human', this report acknowledged that it was not possible to eliminate adverse events from healthcare, but that the system should learn from past experience.[1,2]

There were several recommendations designed to minimise avoidable harm to patients made in the UK report. One of these recommendations was that the experiences of other industries associated with high risk should be examined and, where appropriate, adopted by the National Health Service. The industries being referred to here have been called high-reliability organisations; that is organisations that regard safety concerns as paramount. Civil aviation, offshore oil exploration and nuclear power industries have all been categorised in this way. In these industries it has been established by means of human factors research that, rather than technical performance, human performance is highly significant in the generation and the recovery from adverse events. Human factors is the scientific discipline that is concerned with the interactions between human beings and the environment or system in which they work. This includes investigation of the interactions between humans and machines, the physical design of the work environment and human behaviours in the workplace, e.g. leadership, communication, and decision making. The

Recent Advances in Anaesthesia and Intensive Care 24, ed. J. N. Cashman and R. M. Grounds.
Published by Cambridge University Press. © Cambridge University Press 2007.

European aviation industry collectively called these human behaviours non-technical skills. This term has been adopted in military settings and a number of other industries such as the nuclear power industry, and most recently in healthcare.[3,4]

In the UK, a follow-up implementation report, entitled 'Building a Safer NHS for Patients: Implementing an Organisation with a Memory', was published in 2001.[5] In this report it was highlighted that although patient safety research had been carried out in the UK and other countries, this was not at an advanced stage. Furthermore the report promoted the establishment of a programme of human factors research in healthcare in line with the developments in other industries.

Pre-dating the recommendations of the UK Department of Health safety reports, there is evidence of awareness of the crucial role of non-technical skills in patient safety in the anaesthetic community, and also of lessons having been learnt from other industries. The approach to reduction of hazard and patient safety in anaesthesia has been cited as a model for healthcare.[6,7] This chapter will review the current situation with regard to non-technical skills in anaesthesia, highlighting where there are parallels with other industries.

What are non-technical skills?

Non-technical skills then, are those skills which are required alongside the knowledge and technical skills for any given field of work. In anaesthesia, they can be defined as the behaviours that enhance safety and efficiency that are not directly related to the use of medical expertise, drugs or anaesthetic equipment.[8] They include both social and interpersonal skills (such as team co-ordination, communication, leadership) and also cognitive or mental skills (such as situation awareness and decision-making).

Developments in other industries

Adverse event studies in industries such as aviation have revealed the importance of poor non-technical skills performance in the causation of accidents.[3] More than 30 years before the UK Department of Health safety reports, investigations into adverse events and near misses in aviation had revealed that human error was a major contributor in 70% of accidents.[3] It was argued that improvement in non-technical skills performance could reduce error and therefore reduce the incidence of adverse events.[3] This argument implies that poor non-technical skills performance is implicated in the development of error, and further that good non-technical skills performance can lead to errors being caught, allowing action to be taken to limit their effects. This may capitalise on the fact that individuals regularly correct their own and others' errors in the workplace. From this perspective, it appears that if individuals can be trained to consistently achieve a high level of non-technical skills performance, this will be a key countermeasure to error and adverse event development and to improve management in the workplace.[9]

The aviation industry acknowledged that if maximum safety were to be the prime goal, it was not enough only to ensure that equipment was maintained to a high standard and that flight crews had the appropriate knowledge and technical expertise. Aviation psychology research had shown that it was also necessary to raise individual and organisational awareness of the factors underlying adverse events and near misses, and to devise additional flight crew training for error management. The problems that had been identified related to failures in attention, decision making, leadership and team work. As a result, a research-based training programme known as cockpit resource management was developed in the late 1970s.[9] This programme, now known as crew resource management (CRM), is designed to give participants an understanding of the nature of error in aviation and train them to deal with this more effectively.

Although CRM training was introduced in the 1980s by a number of major airlines, an important stimulus to its widespread adoption was regulatory support in the aviation industry.[10,11] The regulators believed that improved non-technical skills performance would improve safety in the workplace. This led to the sustained development of CRM training and in some countries, e.g. the UK, this training became mandatory.

The transfer of CRM skills from the training environment to the flight deck could not initially be formally assessed. Consequently, a robust method to structure the observation and evaluation of a pilot's CRM skills was required. In Europe, the regulator's advisory group on human factors initiated a project in 1996 to develop a generic method that could be used to evaluate pilots' non-technical skills across Europe.[10,11] This project identified the key skills for pilots from existing systems and in discussion with experienced CRM trainers. Those skills which were observable in practice were ordered into a taxonomy called NOTECHS (non-technical skills), and a definition and behavioural example was provided for each skill element.[10,11] This type of skills set with definitions and exemplar behaviours is called a behavioural marker or rating system. The NOTECHS behavioural marker system was then subjected to extensive experimental and practical evaluations and it was released as a prototype assessment tool. It was then possible for trainers who were qualified to use these tools to give explicit feedback to individuals on their behaviour during training and assessments, and to monitor the development of this skill base in these individuals over time. Versions of the NOTECHS system are now used, by trained assessors, in training and during workplace assessment of pilots in a number of airlines throughout Europe.

The CRM training therefore aims to inform crews of the threats to safety and to enhance the development of behaviours which will reduce error development or act as countermeasures and mitigate against error and adverse events. The skills required to optimise safety behaviour are complementary to the pilots' knowledge and technical skills required to fly a plane.

The CRM training in aviation has been shown to result in improved safety behaviour in the workplace.[12,13] Other high-reliability industries, such as the merchant navy, the offshore oil industry and nuclear power industry, have introduced courses following the same model.[14] Such courses are now increasingly available during anaesthetic training, and are particularly employed in simulation centres.[15]

Developments in anaesthesia

Anaesthesia is conducted in a highly complex work environment. Anaesthetists are required to deal with ill-structured problems in dynamic situations where many variables are operating and there are multiple team members from different professions. Critical events may have to be handled in stressful situations where the stakes are high; there are time pressures, incomplete feedback and shifting goals. It is not surprising that the limits of human performance can be exposed in this setting and evidence is available of poor non-technical skills performance in the development of adverse events and near misses.[16,17,18,19,20,21,22]

To date the overwhelming emphasis in the training of anaesthetists and other healthcare professionals has been directed to supporting the acquisition of knowledge and development of technical skills. This is not to say that anaesthetists have not developed non-technical skills during their training period, but these skills have not been explicitly addressed or encouraged and may be variably acquired.[8]

Anaesthetists and psychologists have investigated the factors contributing to patient safety through adverse event analyses,[17,18] real-life observation studies[20,21,22] and observation in simulation centres.[16,23] Consideration has been given to anaesthetic decision making, the tasks required in anaesthesia and the domain in which anaesthesia is conducted.[24] In addition, there have been steps taken to introduce non-technical skills training into anaesthetic training in many simulation centres, but as yet this is not a required part of the UK anaesthetic curriculum.[16,24,25]

Adverse event analysis

Investigations into adverse events and near misses in anaesthetic practice (and other areas of healthcare) revealed a similar picture to the aviation industry. Investigators have reported that, although contributing factors include technical problems and knowledge issues, in up to 80% of cases the underlying causes of adverse events and near misses were related to non-technical issues such as drug swaps, failures in communication or failure to recognise developing problems resulting in flawed decision making.[17,18]

Real-life observation

In the Shock Trauma Center at the University of Maryland Medical Center there has been a long term project of observation of actual clinical anaesthetic care. The patients' vital signs are captured alongside audio and video recordings of real-life trauma resuscitation, and operating room management. Several of the publications from this group report instances of poor performance of non-technical skills not necessarily in inexperienced trainees but often in expert anaesthetic practitioners. Both social and cognitive issues, such as inadequate communication, problems with decision making and poor awareness of developing problems when cues are missed, are described.[20,21,22,23]

Simulation centre observation

Simulation training has steadily grown in anaesthesia since the mid 1980s.[15] Trainers working at simulation centres have now observed many hundreds of anaesthetic trainees in critical scenarios. As investigation into adverse events and real-life observational studies suggest, although problems with knowledge and technical skills are regularly in evidence, many deficiencies in non-technical performance are also observed.[8,16,25]

Crew Resource Management training in anaesthesia

Howard and colleagues were aware of parallels between anaesthesia and aviation such as the need to operate in complex environments, the close interaction with technology and the significant influence of human error in the development of adverse events. In 1990, they reported the development of a course called Anaesthesia Crisis Resource Management (ACRM) which was based on the principles of CRM.[16] The course was run in a mock-up of an operating theatre and used a high-fidelity patient simulator to expose participants to a number of critical clinical incidents. With video assistance, the participants were then debriefed not only on their knowledge and technical skills, but also on the non-technical aspects of their performance. An ACRM programme typically takes place on three separate days run over three years of the anaesthesia syllabus. The course has been positively received by participants, who report that it supports their safe practice of anaesthesia.[24] The world-wide spread of computer-driven patient simulators has served to further increase interest in non-technical skills in anaesthesia. Courses based on the ACRM course are now taught across the world and are a required part of training for anaesthetic practitioners in some countries.[15] Other training courses have been developed on a wide range of simulator devices, from full operating simulations to lower fidelity computer-based simulations.[8,15] As with the development of CRM in aviation, in order to support the debriefing of anaesthetic participants in simulator courses, trainers sought a framework for identification and assessment of the non-technical aspects of performance they were witnessing and turned to behavioural marker systems. In 2001, a review of the non-technical skills behavioural marker systems used in anaesthesia revealed that there was no common system in use and further that those in practice had been primarily derived from aviation.[8,27]

Although the information and tools for non-technical skills training from other domains of work can be useful as models, they should not be directly extrapolated.[3] Key differences in the domains may render these tools inappropriate. Examples of differences between aviation and anaesthesia include:

- In aviation although the number of adverse events is probably many times greater than the number of events causing accidents, the frequency of these events are considered to be far less frequent than in anaesthesia. Significant adverse events have been reported in up to 5% of anaesthetics, even where performed by experts.[28]

- In contrast with aviation and other industries, leadership is often ill defined in the operating room. There are several professional groups (e.g. nursing, anaesthesia, surgery) and although the overall goal of each is safe progress of the patient through the perioperative period, each group has differing areas of knowledge, skill and responsibility for the patient. This may result in disagreements about the overall priority for the patient and what the greatest priorities are for patient care at any given time.[25]

- Perhaps one of the greatest differences between aviation and anaesthesia is the contrast between a plane and the patient. Unlike aircraft, which are designed and built to work in a standardised manner, each patient is a highly complex system where there are multiple poorly understood interactions. In addition each patient has a unique set of problems and pathophysiology, and the impact of anaesthesia and surgery on this is imperfectly understood.[29]

With this concern in mind, a project called the 'anaesthetists' non-technical skills project' (ANTS) was begun in 1999 in order to define the skills particular to anaesthesia. The goal of the project was to develop a behavioural marker system which would be grounded empirically in anaesthetic practice.

Development of an anaesthetists' non-technical skills taxonomy

A literature review of the role of non-technical skills in anaesthesia by the team undertaking this project had concluded that it was clear that non-technical skills played a central role in anaesthetic practice.[8] However, it was not possible from the review to identify a full list of which skills were important and how these were actually used in anaesthetic practice.

Behavioural marker systems are context specific and should be developed for the domain in which they will be used.[4] Not only will the key behaviours vary across professions but they can vary in different national cultures within the same profession.[9] Those evaluating the impact of CRM training in the aviation industry became aware that what worked well in North America did not necessarily work well in other parts of the world. The anaesthetists' non-technical skills (ANTS) project, sponsored by NHS Education for Scotland, aimed to develop a validated behavioural marker system for the identification and assessment of non-technical skills in anaesthesia from first principles.

A team of industrial psychologists and clinical anaesthetists collaborated in the project. A method similar to that used in other industries was adopted to identify the relevant skills; adverse event and near miss analysis; attitudinal surveys; cognitive task interviews of experts in the field and observation of anaesthesia in both the simulator and real life.[30]

The resulting system is hierarchical with four skill categories at the highest level (Task management, Team working, Situation awareness and Decision making; Fig. 12.1). These categories are then further divided into 15 elements. Each element has linked observable example behaviours of both good and poor practice (Fig. 12.2). It is important to note that the system was not designed to be fully exhaustive and is limited to the principal skills

Fig. 12.1 The ANTS system.

Category	Element
Task management	Planning and preparing Prioritising Providing and maintaining standards Identifying and utilising resources
Team working	Co-ordinating activities with team members Exchanging information Using authority and assertiveness Assessing capabilities Supporting others
Situation awareness	Gathering information Recognising and understanding Anticipating
Decision making	Identifying options Balancing risks and selecting options Re-evaluating

Fig. 12.2 Example of behavioural markers for the element: co-ordinating activities with team members.

Behavioural markers for good practice	Behavioural markers for poor practice
• Confirms roles and responsibilities of team members	• Does not co-ordinate with surgeons and other groups
• Discusses care with surgeons or colleagues	• Relies too much on familiarity of team for getting things done
• Considers requirements of others before acting	• Intervenes without informing/involving others
• Co-operates with others to achieve goals	• Does not involve team in tasks

which can be identified through observable behaviour. Hence stress management and communication are not included because stress management is difficult to observe and communication is frequently the means by which the other skills are inferred.

Assessment of an individual can be made at both the element and category levels. A rating scale was developed alongside the system. This was used during the ANTS experimental evaluation and user trials.[30,31] This has four points for describing level of performance with an additional option for non-observed skills (Fig. 12.3). The non-observed option is available for use in circumstances when it is not appropriate for an element to be demonstrated.

The ANTS project was the first empirically derived and validated investigation of the non-technical skills required for a healthcare profession. The

Fig. 12.3 ANTS system rating options.

Rating label	Description
4 = good	Performance was of a consistently high standard, enhancing patient safety; it could be used as a positive example for others
3 = acceptable	Performance was of a satisfactory standard but could be improved
2 = marginal	Performance indicated cause for concern, considerable improvement is needed
1 = poor	Performance endangered or potentially endangered patient safety, serious remediation is required
not observed	Skill could not be observed in this scenario

resulting taxonomy can provide a basis for the training of anaesthetic non-technical skills which are observable for the individual both in theatre settings and during sessions at a simulation centre. Use of ANTS offers the opportunity for assessors trained in the system to give specific feedback to anaesthetic trainees on the behaviours that have been observed. However, if an overall assessment of performance for each category or element is the goal, there remains the significant problem of rating across a prolonged period or a whole anaesthetic case. Over even a short period of time in any anaesthetic case, examples of both good and less good performance attributable to the same element or category may be seen. This issue can cause difficulties in rating overall performance, and has been previously reported when assessing both technical and non-technical elements of performance.[32]

Non-technical skills training developments in anaesthesia

The ANTS system was developed to allow non-technical skills training for anaesthetists to be structured. From the interest expressed to the authors since information on ANTS version one was published in 2003,[30] it seems clear that many anaesthetic trainers across the world were eager for such a training tool. By 2006 the system had been translated into Hebrew and German and a booklet published on the system had been requested by anaesthetists across the world including Australia, New Zealand, USA, Canada, Germany, the Netherlands and Switzerland (the German translation and ANTS booklet can be accessed at www.abdn.ac.uk/iprc/ANTS). The CRM-type courses have become widespread, wherever there are anaesthetic simulation centres, and many of the requests for information and reports of use of ANTS have come from trainers associated with these centres (personal communication).

Yee and colleagues used the ANTS behavioural marker system in a Canadian simulation centre to prospectively investigate the effect of repeated simulation sessions with video debriefing on the non-technical skills of anaesthetic trainees.[26] They noted that previous studies had demonstrated improvement of technical ability and knowledge with such repeated exposure to simulation. In this study, raters trained in the ANTS system assessed the non-technical skills of the participants at each session. The study confirmed that like other aspects of performance, with specific structured training, trainees' performance of non-technical skills can improve with repeated simulation training.

Yee and colleagues commented that some of the categories and elements of the ANTS system are linked to medical knowledge and expertise (e.g. providing and maintaining standards). They highlight that the performance of non-technical skills can therefore be influenced by the subject's medical knowledge. In use of the system for assessment purposes it would be important to select cases that were appropriate to a particular trainee's stage of development.

Rosenstock and colleagues also draw attention to the link between medical knowledge and some of the non-technical skill elements in the ANTS system.[33] They performed a retrospective analysis of unanticipated difficult airway management, and found the ANTS system useful as a framework for assessing the performance of non-technical skills. They looked for evidence of use of three of the four ANTS categories (task management, situation awareness and decision making). Data were collected from questionnaires and semi-structured interviews shortly after each difficult airway management event. Where there were non-technical skills problems in dealing with the clinical event, they reported that mainly task management skills were impaired. They suggested that a significant underlying contributing factor might be the lack of a uniform standard or guideline for difficult airway management in Scandinavia which resulted in limited knowledge and consequently poor task management.

Although the ANTS system has been welcomed as the first such assessment tool grounded in the domain, some criticisms have been raised. Rall and Gaba argue that the ANTS tool assumes that the non-technical skills are generic and context free and therefore does not differentiate between those skills which might be required in particular scenarios or clinical settings.[15] Highlighting that the intent of ANTS is to score only the skills which can be observed, Rall and Gaba note that with use of this system, relevant personal factors such as stress management may not be considered.[15]

Integration of explicit non-technical skills training, with or without use of the ANTS system, into routine anaesthetic training is still at an early stage.

The ANTS project provides insight into key non-technical skills required in the domain. When training is introduced and how best to support the development of these skills has still to be established.[34]

Where there are simulation centres, ACRM-type training is increasingly common. However it is not a mandatory part of the anaesthetic syllabus for all, although it is interesting to note that in the USA one insurer has offered a reduced malpractice premium for any anaesthesia member of staff who has undergone ACRM training.[35] This has resulted in the development of a continuing professional development ACRM course at the Harvard Centre for medical simulation for career-grade anaesthesiologists.[35]

The ANTS system was designed not only with simulation centres in mind, but also for training in the workplace.[30] In the UK, the ANTS system has been presented to the Education Strategy Committee of the Royal College of Anaesthetists. This led to a pilot investigation of introduction of the system into general clinical training being sponsored. The method adopted in the pilot investigation was to run a one-day introductory course, facilitated by one of the anaesthetists involved in developing the ANTS system, to local enthusiasts in a number of UK training centres. It was hoped that if these enthusiasts could gain confidence in use of the system then they would be in a position to further cascade training in the use of the system within their own departments. This could allow non-technical skills to be explicitly identified during routine training and feedback to be given on trainee performance.

Trainers within any cascade system require support if they are to be successful in their mission.[36] This includes support for the development of the cascade trainers themselves and training materials for the proposed training. As these tools are still in development it is perhaps not surprising that this pilot introduction has not yet resulted in established use of the ANTS system as an explicit training tool in the clinical area in the UK.

Perhaps it should not be surprising that, despite significant progress in non-technical skills training in anaesthesia, there still seems to be much development to come. In aviation, CRM training has evolved through several generations over almost 30 years of development.[9] From the second generation of CRM it was agreed that the training would evolve so that it was fully embedded into the flight training and operation rather than a stand-alone topic. Simulator training has been coupled with in-flight assessment and feedback from trained raters for both trainee and qualified pilots.[9,12] In addition the training has extended to include the whole flight team and not only the pilots. This was reflected by the change of title from cockpit to crew resource management.[9]

Similarly in healthcare there have been efforts to provide training for the whole operative team.[37,38,39] Moorthy and team have described extending the use of surgical simulation beyond the training of technical skills to include non-technical skills including team working. However although the anaesthetist was part of the team the scenario and training was focused on providing feedback to the surgeons rather than the whole team.[37] They are now working on scenario development, which will require non-technical skills performance and therefore permit feedback to all members of the operative team including anaesthetists, nurses and surgeons.[38] They report working on the development of performance measures for the whole team. From an aviation framework, Helmreich and Schaefer derived a model for operating-room assessment of the whole team.[39] Rather than individual performance feedback it is the whole team's performance which is assessed and team communications and interactions are explored. Whether it is for the training of individuals or the training of teams, in order to best develop non-technical skills it is essential that they are incorporated into the curriculum, explicitly and in a structured manner.[21,38,40]

Non-technical skills in related disciplines

A similar series of investigations into the crucial non-technical skills for surgeons during the operative period has followed the ANTS project. Unsurprisingly, a review of the literature suggests that non-technical skills in addition to technical skills are necessary to maintain high levels of surgical performance.[41] Following a similar empirical approach to the ANTS project, a prototype behavioural marker system of non-technical skills for surgeons (NOTSS) has been developed and has undergone preliminary evaluation.[42] Training courses in surgical non-technical skills have been run by the Royal College of Surgeons of Edinburgh and further courses are currently planned.

Regarding the field of intensive care, Reader and colleagues considered that many of the principles which related to performance and safety in anaesthesia were also relevant to the intensive care unit.[43] They conducted a review of the existing critical incident literature from intensive care, and found that a large proportion of the identified contributory factors which underlay the incidents could be attributed to one of the skill categories from the anaesthetists' non-technical skills system. They suggested that although this appeared to be a good starting point, because the intensive care setting presents its own unique challenges, further human factors research would be required to better understand the non-technical skills which are important in this environment.[43]

Other acute hospital specialty groups that have shown interest in the development of non-technical skills training at various presentations and workshops on ANTS include obstetrics, acute general medicine and emergency medicine.

Summary

Good performance of non-technical skills has been shown to be important in both the reduction of error and in mitigating against the effects of error in many sectors where safety is a major concern. This is also the case for healthcare in general and anaesthesia in particular, where patient safety is a concern and training in non-technical skills has previously not been explicit. Non-technical skills developments in anaesthesia have been significant. They include: simulation-centre training, based on the CRM principles first developed in the aviation industry, and human factors research into the non-technical skills important for anaesthesia, to assist with the skills identification and give feedback to trainees. However, although these are explicit developments there is still much progress required for non-technical skills training to be embedded into the anaesthetic training curriculum in both simulated and clinical settings. There is a requirement for the development of training materials and training of the trainers.

A further research programme is in the process of evaluating a prototype non-technical skills behavioural marker system for surgeons in the operating room. If these systems were to be properly integrated into the curricula of each specialty with the appropriate training of trainers and development of supporting materials, this could offer the exciting opportunity of team training with targeted feedback for individual operating team members some time in the future.

References

1. Department of Health. *An Organization with a Memory*. London: Department of Health, 2000.
2. Kohn LT, Corrigan JM, Donaldson MS (eds.). *To Err is Human: Building a Safer Health System*. Washington, DC: Institute of Medicine, 1999.
3. Helmreich RL. On error management: lessons from aviation. *BMJ* 2000; **320**: 781–5.
4. Klampfer B, Flin R, Helmreich RL, *et al*. Enhancing performance in high-risk environments: Recommendations for the use of behavioural markers; www.abdn.ac.UK/iprc/papers%20reports/Ants/GIHRE21_rec_for_use_of_beh_markers.pdf
5. Department of Health. *Building a Safer NHS for Patients: Implementing an Organisation with a Memory*. London: Department of Health, 2001.

6. Cooper JB, Gaba DM. No myth: anesthesia is a model for addressing patient safety. *Anesthesiology* 2002; **97**: 1335–7.
7. Gaba DM. Anaesthesiology as a model for patient safety in health care. *BMJ* 2000; **320**: 785–8.
8. Fletcher GL, McGeorge P, Flin R, Glavin R, Maran N. The role of non-technical skills in anaesthesia: a review of current literature. *Br J Anaesth* 2002; **88**: 418–29.
9. Helmreich RL, Merritt AC, Wilhelm JA. The evolution of crew resource management training in commercial aviation. *Int J Aviat Psychol* 1999; **9**: 19–32.
10. Flin R, Goeters K-M, Hörmann H-J, *et al.* Development of the NOTECHS (non-technical skills) system for assessing pilots' CRM skills. *Hum Factors Aerospace Saf* 2003; **3**: 95–117.
11. O'Connor P, Hörmann H-J, Flin R, Lodge M, Goeters K-M. The JARTEL Group. Developing a method for evaluating crew resource management skills: a European perspective. *Int J Aviat Psychol* 2002; **12**: 263–85.
12. Goeters KM. Evaluation of the effects of CRM training by the assessment of non-technical skills under LOFT. *Hum Factors Aerospace Saf* 2002; **2**: 71–86.
13. Salas E, Wilson KA, Burke CS. Does crew resource management work? An update, an extension, and some critical needs. *Hum Factors* 2006; **48**: 392–412.
14. Flin R, O'Connor P, Mearns K. Crew resource management: improving team work in high-reliability industries. *Team Perform Manage* 2002; **8**: 68–78.
15. Rall M, Gaba DM. Patient simulators. In *Miller's Anesthesia*, 6th edn. Philadelphia, PA: Churchill Livingstone, 2005; pp. 3073–103.
16. Howard SK, Gaba DM, Fish KJ, Yang G, Sarnquist FH. Anesthesia crisis resource management training: teaching anesthesiologists to handle critical incidents. *Aviat Space Environ Med* 1992; **63**: 763–70.
17. Cooper JB, Newbower RS, Long CD, McPeek B. Preventable anesthesia mishaps: a study of human factors. *Anesthesiology* 1978; **49**: 399–406.
18. Williamson JA, Webb RK, Sellen A, Runciman WB, Van Der Walt JH. Human failure: an analysis of 2000 incident reports. *Anaesth Intensive Care* 1993; **21**: 678–83.
19. Bogner M, (ed.) *Misadventures in Health Care*. Mahwah, NJ: LEA; 2004.
20. Xiao Y, Mackenzie CF, the LOTAS Group. Decision making in dynamic environments: fixation errors and their causes. In *Proceedings of the 39th Annual Meeting of the Human Factors and Ergonomics Society*. Santa Monica, CA: Human Factors and Ergonomics Society, 1995; pp. 469–73.
21. Xiao Y, Mackenzie CF. Collaboration in complex medical systems. In *Collaborative Crew Performance in Complex Operational Systems*. NATO Human Factors and Medicine Symposium, April 20–24, 1998. Neuilly sur Seire: NATO, 1998; 4–1 to 4–10.
22. Xiao Y, Hunter WA, McKenzie CF, *et al.* Task complexity in emergency medical care and its implications for team coordination. LOTAS group. Level-one trauma anaesthesia simulation. *Hum Factors* 1996; **38**: 636–43.
23. Xiao Y, Mackenzie CF, Patey R, the LOTAS Group. Team co-ordination and breakdowns in a real-life stressful environment. In *Proceedings of the Human*

Factors and Ergonomics Society 42nd Annual Meeting. Santa Monica, CA: Human Factors and Ergonomics Society, 1998; pp. 186–90.

24. Kyle HT, Gaba DM. Safe passage: using simulation to teach patient safety. *Clin Teach* 2005; **2**: 37–41.

25. Rall M, Gaba DM. Human performance and patient safety. In *Miller's Anesthesia*, 6th edn. Philadelphia, PA: Churchill Livingstone, 2005; pp. 3021–72.

26. Yee B, Naik VN, Joo HS, *et al.* Non-technical skills in anesthesia crisis management with repeated exposure to simulation-based education. *Anesthesiology* 2005; **103**: 241–8.

27. Fletcher G, Flin R, McGeorge P. *Review of Behavioural Marker Systems in Anaesthesia*. Workpackage 2 Report, 2000; accessible at www.abdn.ac.uk/iprc/ANTS.

28. Forrest JB, Cahalan MK, Rehder K. Multicenter study of general anesthesia II. Results. *Anesthesiology* 1990; **72**: 262–8.

29. Gaba DM, Maxwell M, DeAnda A. Anesthetic mishaps: breaking the chain of accident evolution. *Anesthesiology* 1987; **66**: 670–6.

30. Fletcher G, Flin R, McGeorge P, *et al.* Anaesthetists' Non-technical Skills (ANTS): evaluation of a behavioural marker system. *Br J Anaesth* 2003; **90**: 580–8.

31. Patey R, Flin R, Fletcher G, Maran N, Glavin R. *Anaesthetists' non-technical skills (ANTS). Advances in Patient Safety: From Research to Implementation*. Special Edition 2004. US Agency for Healthcare Research and Quality.

32. Gaba DM, Howard SK, Flanagan B, *et al.* Assessment of clinical performance during simulated crises using both technical and behavioural ratings. *Anesthesiology* 1998; **89**: 8–18.

33. Rosenstock C, Hansen EG, Kristensen MS, Rasmussen LS, Skak C. Østergaard D. Qualitative analysis of unanticipated difficult airway management. *Acta Anaesthesiol Scand* 2006; **50**: 290–7.

34. Glavin R, Maran N. Integrating human factors into the medical curriculum. *Med Educ* (Supplement) 2003; **37**: 59–64.

35. Blum RH, Raemer DB, Carroll JS, *et al.* Crisis resources management training for an anaesthesia faculty: a new approach to continuing education. *Med Educ* 2004; **38**: 45–55.

36. Hayes D. Cascade training and teachers' professional development. *Engl Lang Teach J* 2000; **54**: 135–45.

37. Moorthy K, Munz Y, Adams S, Pandey Y, Darzi A. A human factors analysis of technical and team skills during procedural simulations. *Br J Surg* 2004: **90** (Suppl. 1): 88–9.

38. Moorthy K, Vincent C, Darzi A. Simulation-based training. *Br Med J* 2005; **330**: 493–4.

39. Helmreich RL, Schaefer H-G, Sexton JB. *Operating Room Checklist Aerospace Crew Resource Project Technical Report 95–4*. Austin, TX: University of Texas, 1995.

40. Davies J. Team communication in the operating room. *Acta Anaesthesiol Scand* 2005; **49**: 898–901.

41. Yule S, Flin R, Paterson-Brown S, Maran N. Non-technical skills for surgeons in the operating room: A review of the literature. *Surgery* 2006; **139**: 140–9.

42. Yule S, Flin R, Paterson-Brown S, Maran N, Rowley D. Development of a rating system for surgeons' non-technical skills. *Med Educ* 2006; **40**: 1098–104.

43. Reader R, Flin R, Lauche K, Cuthbertson BH. Non-technical skills in the intensive care unit. *Br J Anaesth* 2006; **96**: 551–9.

Peter Dieckmann and Marcus Rall

Simulators in anaesthetic training to enhance patient safety

Simulation is revolutionising the education and training of anaesthetists all over the world and is a significant contributor to enhancing patient safety. Anaesthesiology is once again emphasising its role as a pioneering discipline for increasing patient safety.[1,2] Different forms of simulators are available in many countries and new types of simulators are being further developed.[3,4,5,6] Recently the field has also advanced in conceptual terms with new and creative ideas for using these advanced technical tools. Simulators are used in educational settings, for research, and for assessment. The traditional centre-based simulations are now supplemented by mobile '*in situ*' simulation training,[7] bringing simulation to work places.[8] New instructors can choose from a variety of courses and other resources for learning the craft and the art of conducting simulations.[9,10,11,12,13,14,15]

The introduction of simulation, especially with video-based debriefing, contributed considerably to the discussing of human factor theories in the medical domain. In anaesthesia this process was pioneered by Cooper and the group led by Gaba and Howard with their concept of crisis resource management (CRM (c.f. crew resource management, Ch. 12)).[16,17,18,19,20,21,22] The CRM-based simulation course model made its way around the globe. Simulation worked as a very powerful tool to make healthcare professionals aware of the impact of human error and how to deal with human limitations, and how best to use unique human capabilities in order to reduce errors, detect problems early and to take effective teamwork countermeasures to ensure patient safety.

Human and systems errors are seen as root causes in about 70% of incidents and accidents.[16,21,22,23,24,25,26,27] Simulation has great potential for

Recent Advances in Anaesthesia and Intensive Care 24, ed. J. N. Cashman and R. M. Grounds.
Published by Cambridge University Press. © Cambridge University Press 2007.

increasing patient safety.[28,29] If simulation is used more widely, *'firsts'* on living patients will be greatly reduced; that is, healthcare professionals will have learned the necessary skills and practised clinical procedures to a sufficient level before performing them on a patient for the first time. This is a revolution regarding the traditional method of apprenticeship-style of learning by doing (and making mistakes during) invasive procedures on living patients. In the same way healthcare providers should, through recurrent team simulations of all expected problems, become better prepared for the prevention and handling of crisis situations, thus increasing emergency prevention and preparedness. As a research tool simulation will enhance the current knowledge and methods for safe healthcare by providing a unique realistic laboratory to analyse and improve the practice of care, to address its related problems (e.g. fatigue), and to improve teaching and learning.

In this chapter we define the important concepts for using simulators and simulations, describe different formats of simulator use, differentiate ideas about simulation-based learning relevant to simulation, discuss challenges for simulator instructors, and describe future developments. We focus on mannikin-based patient simulators for their educational use but touch briefly on different forms of simulation and other uses.

Defining simulators and simulations

In any discussion of simulators and simulations it is important to agree on basic definitions and in particular the difference between the words 'simula*tor*' and 'simula*tion*'.[30] We present a broad view of these terms to include aspects important for using simulators and simulations that go beyond the technical device (see Fig. 13.1).[6]

Simulator versus simulation

The 'simulator' provides the (physically represented) *interfaces* that allow the users to interact with the simulation. In anaesthesia manikin-based, screen-based, or part-task trainers are commonly used. In this chapter we will focus on full-scale manikin-based simulators and simulations.

The word 'simulation' has at least two meanings. One meaning refers to the *simulation mechanism*, which is a means (mostly software, but possibly also pieces of paper, and even thoughts) of representing physiological processes. Based on an increasing level of automation, there are three different types of software-based simulation mechanisms: the mechanism can be manually controlled (physiological changes are entered

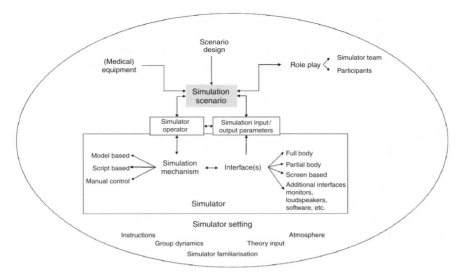

Fig. 13.1 The 'anatomy' and surroundings of simulation and simulators.

individually), script-based (several parameters can be linked together using a scripting language) or model based (a mathematical physiology model is used to compute the necessary and interrelated changes of different parameters). In any case the simulation mechanism integrates inputs and generates output parameters that are presented via different output interfaces to participants and to the simulator team running the scenario. The person actually manipulating the simulation mechanism is called the *simulator operator*.[6]

The second meaning of the word 'simulation' concerns a *simulation scenario*, which is an enactment of a clinical case, a specific problem or a task, using the patient simulator, the simulator room, medical equipment, role players etc.[31] Such additional elements are typically intended to enhance the perceived realism of the scenario (psychological simulation fidelity),[32,33] although these elements can also reduce psychological fidelity if they are constructed or implemented inadequately. It is important to note that increased simulation fidelity does not necessarily mean higher educational impact and relevance of scenarios. Simulation fidelity in its technical, social, functional or other facets must be tailored to the goals of the simulation.[14,15]

Connections between simulation mechanism and simulation scenario

The connections between the simulation mechanism and the simulation scenario are established via interfaces for input (from the scenario to the simulation mechanism) and output (from the simulation mechanism to the scenario). The patient manikin provides both types of interfaces (e.g. input: IV lines, body checks; output: thorax movements, loudspeakers for breathing sounds). Other output interfaces are the vital signs monitor (e.g. ECG, blood pressure), the simulator operator, and other actors who role play the patient or verbally simulate aspects that cannot (yet) be simulated otherwise (e.g. changes of skin colour, temperature of the simulated patient). Note that, in Fig. 13.1, we have termed both the actions of the simulator team and the participants *role play* according to Mann:[34] even if participants are asked to *be themselves* they act under artificial circumstances during a simulation scenario.

Sensors built into the manikin can automatically provide some input according to participants' actions (e.g. drug recognition systems or sensors for ventilation frequency and tidal volume). However, for many participant actions, the simulator operator is needed as an interpreter: he or she observes what participants do and translates these actions into meaningful input for the simulation mechanism (e.g. administering a drug by selecting it in the software application or adjusting physiological parameters). In some cases the simulator operator modifies those inputs (e.g. changing the injected dosage of the drug) in the attempt to achieve specific goals of the simulation scenario. For example, in many courses for healthcare students physiological responses are slowed down or simulated as less severe to give the students time to think and solve the problem instead of learning that patients die 'realistically'. In these cases the simulator operator should be seen as part of the simulation mechanism.

Simulation is more than having a simulator: the setting concept

The simulation scenario is just one part of the simulator setting. A simulation-based training course has several other modules including theory inputs, instructions on how to use the simulator, and debriefings after the scenario.[14] Reference to Fig. 13.1 will assist simulator teams to get a clearer understanding of what to improve if scenarios are problematic by analysing which element, or connection between elements, in the structure caused a problem.

There are a variety of different simulators and different simulations which can be used in different settings and ways. Also we agree with Gaba who has emphasised the need to consider the context in which simulation as a technical device is used (see Table 13.1).[7] We think that another important category should be added to his dimensions: the integration of simulation into the organisation, the profession, or even the society. For example in Denmark it is a requirement to take part in simulation when specialising in anaesthesia, whilst in Germany simulation is still a *'nice to have'* feature.

Table 13.1 The dimensions of simulation application.

Purpose and aims of the simulation activity
Unit of participation in the simulation
Experience level of participants
Health care domain in which simulation is applied
Health care discipline of personnel participating in the simulation
Type of knowledge, skill, attitudes, or behaviours addressed in simulation
Age of the patient being simulated
Technology applicable or required for the simulation
Site of simulation participation
Extent of direct participation of simulation
Feedback method accompanying simulation
Organisational, professional, societal embedding of simulation*

*Additional category, not mentioned by Gaba.[7]
Source: Gaba,[7] and Dieckmann.[14]

Looking closer at the aims and objectives with which simulators and simulations are used in anaesthesia, one can distinguish between educational, research-related, and assessment-related purposes. In the following we focus on the educational use of simulators.

Different educational uses of simulators and simulations

Basic courses for healthcare students

During basic education the focus of simulator use lies on medical/technical knowledge (e.g. physiology, pharmacokinetics, pharmacodynamics) and skills (e.g. placing IV lines, intubating, approaching unconscious patients). However, we think an early exposure to human factors concepts and crisis resource management is important for healthcare students to foster a cultural change within the medical field. During simulation, students get one of the first opportunities to actually interact with 'a patient' in a responsible way and a safe environment, and participants value this opportunity very highly.[35] This way healthcare students can acknowledge that medical competency comprises more than declarative knowledge – that, however, is still predominantly the focus of the initial training.

Continuous medical educations: crisis resource management (CRM)

Among the most promising educational uses of simulations and simulators are courses for crisis resource management with video-assisted debriefing. These courses do make the best use of the unique properties of simulator settings. They allow for replicating the complex interplay of humans, technology, and organisation that is relevant for (patient)

Table 13.2 Key points of crisis resource management (CRM).

Know the environment
Anticipate and plan
Call for help early
Exercise leadership and followership
Distribute the workload
Mobilise all available resources
Communicate effectively
Use all available information
Prevent and manage fixation errors
Cross (double) check
Use cognitive aids
Re-evaluate repeatedly
Use good teamwork
Allocate attention wisely
Set priorities dynamically

Source: Rall and Gaba.[25]

---

safety.[22,25,36] Role players do take part in simulation scenarios to make the scene more lively but in addition can also be scripted to present interpersonal challenges that participants can hardly learn to deal with in other settings. Equipment problems can be built into scenarios, as well as organisational issues, like time pressure. On the one hand the specific management of problems can be enhanced, for example using the ABC algorithm or treating anaphylactic shock. On the other hand more general principles of team work and individual performance can be addressed. In many centres the principles of crisis resource management (CRM) are used as the gold-standard (see Table 13.2).[19,25] Being a safe environment, simulations allow for 'retrivialising' human error in medicine. In contrast to the clinical setting, there are no patients endangered during simulation. Taking the burden of tragic consequences off from learners helps them to analyse, reflect, and possibly optimise, their habits in treating patients.

The scenario offers the possibility for experiences and experiential learning and the debriefing offers a secure frame for reflection, discussion and integration of these experiences. Modern audio/video systems allow for recording different perspectives at the same time (Fig. 13.2). During facilitated discussions, strengths and weaknesses of the medical/technical as well as CRM performance can be analysed and alternative approaches discussed.[37] Exchanging perspectives allows participants to broaden their view on patient safety. Facilitating debriefing often poses some burden on instructors who have little experience with such interactive methods, emphasising the benefit of engaging in thorough instructor training before working with simulators and simulations.[38]

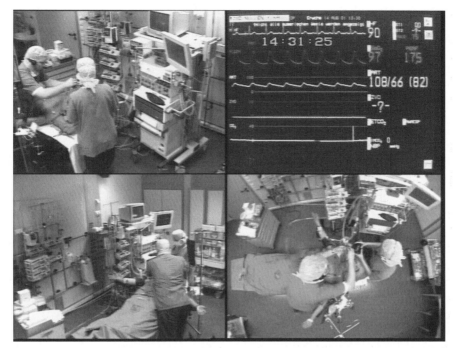

Fig. 13.2 Different perspectives recorded from one simulation scenario using modern audio/video recording.

Continuous medical educations: special medical technical topics

Modern patient simulators allow for simulating various aspects that interest anaesthesiologists, like many forms of the difficult airway,[39] circulation problems, and other diseases, complications, and critical incidents. They are also suitable for general emergency response and code trainings. The simulation scenarios can be used to connect theory and practice in a way that is hardly achievable in other settings. Short lectures and workshops can be used for preparation and aftermaths of the scenarios, delivering pieces of information on the spot. Complex scenarios might also help participants discover learning needs.

Mobile 'in situ' training

A recently growing training format is the concept of the mobile 'in situ'[7,8,40] simulation. The idea is to bring the simulator to where participants actually work and to train together those who work together. This approach has been used in various healthcare settings, such as cardiac-catheter laboratories (Fig. 13.3), air-rescue jets and helicopters, ambulance cars, and dental practices. In contrast to centre-based simulator trainings,

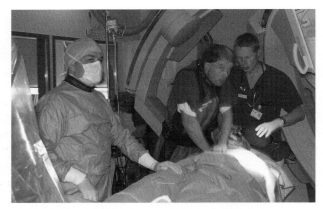

Fig. 13.3 *'In situ'* mobile simulation in a heart catheterisation laboratory.

participants in mobile simulation courses do know the environment in which the case is simulated and need less familiarisation with the surroundings. They can concentrate more on training contents. However, acting within their own organisation within simulation changes many processes, perceptions, and interpretations. Learning is a different activity[41] than working, even if conducted in the same location. Activities can be distinguished by basic motives (i.e. working versus learning) and provide the framework for the goal-oriented actions of which they are composed. So, even if providing anaesthesia in the simulator looks similar to the clinical environment, it is still a different activity as it follows different basic motives. These differences need to be accounted for in the training concepts.

During mobile courses, simulation becomes more than training – it often serves as a kind of organisational development. Many of the relevant agents of organisational improvements are present during *in situ* simulation courses, facilitating organisational improvements. *In situ* simulation also helps in questioning existing habits. Simulator instructors can almost become consultants who help take a second look at what might have been taken for granted for a long time.

However, conducting mobile courses also poses some challenges, especially for the simulator team. The instructors do need a good familiarisation with the local characteristics. Instructors need to interpret local jargon; for example, recognising that *'calling the second floor'* is an appropriate call for help in a given organisation. Further, a mobile simulation course is integrated into existing group dynamics and is influenced by alliances, coalitions, or hierarchy within the group of participants. Setting up an *'in situ'* training with video-assisted debriefing is a considerable logistical and technical challenge, requiring several cameras and microphones

(Fig. 13.4). However, from our experience the benefit is easily worth the effort (see Table 13.3).

Presentations and conference workshops

Another type of educational use of simulators comprises demonstrations of the technology at meetings and conventions. Such demonstrations focus on different contents, like demonstrating typical crisis resource management scenarios or particularities in using a specific (type) of drug or equipment (e.g. different tools for airway management, infusion pumps). Such presentations are often meant to spread the idea of simulation more broadly.

Different ideas of simulation-based learning

Having the simulator available is only one part of conducting educational simulations. Maybe even more important are the educational concepts that guide their use. A basic distinction can be made between knowledge, skills, and attitudes, which all together comprise (medical) competency. *Knowledge* comprises declarative aspects like facts, pieces of information. *Skills* comprise procedural aspects, like sequencing of tasks and applying knowledge. Skills also have a sensumotoric part requiring eye–hand co-ordination in difficult movements, for example during intubation. *Attitudes* should be seen in a broad sense, for example also containing the values and beliefs a person has. They influence the interpretation of a specific situation, but also the decisions about how to act within this situation. The different teaching goals are related closely to the ideas about learning in simulation. Different approaches can be distinguished.

The '*learn it here and do it there*' approach

This idea focuses on drill-and-practice type learning. Participants are asked to perform and repeat a specific procedure or skill in the simulation until they can perform it up to a reasonable level. The focus lies on sensumotoric and procedural skills. It is hoped that this acquired skill can be transferred to the clinical setting. Practising placing an IV line with a so-called 'part-task trainer' could reduce the learning time with real patients. This type of simulation-based learning requires high physical simulation fidelity, as sensumotoric aspects can be learned better if the simulation replicates the characteristics of the human body as closely as possible, changing the required manoeuvres as little as possible.

Table 13.3 Indications, advantages and challenges of mobile 'in situ' simulator training.

Indications	Advantages	Challenges
• Participants are not 'mobile' (e.g. hard to free from clinical duties). • The environment is hard to simulate (e.g. space constrictions, noise, variations). • Wish to 'test' the clinical environment and the response system.	• Less travel time (two or three instructors travel, not 12 to 14 participants). • Often it is less effort to provide mobile simulation than to replicate the relevant environment – mock-ups are less mobile/flexible. • Application of what was learned during simulation might be easier because of higher practical value of training. • Participants can work in their known environment, often increasing relevance of training. • Participants of in situ training can become a change hot spot – initiating and implementing many improvements. • Training and organisational development are closely related, and feedback from training can help to improve processes.	• Instructors need familiarisation with local conditions and practices. • Existing group dynamics might disturb the training (touching taboos, alliances, etc.). • Mobile equipment is expensive and needs good insurance, especially because equipment is strained considerably during transportation. • Instructors need to travel a lot. • The instructors need good logistical support on site, which is not always easy to organise.

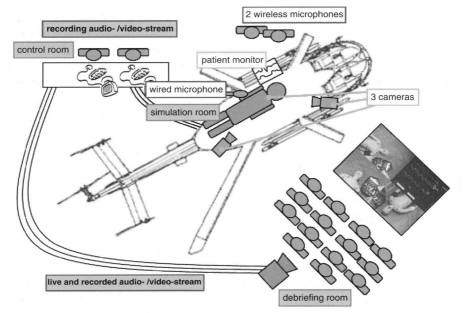

Fig. 13.4 Schematic technical set-up of mobile 'in situ' simulation in a helicopter.

The 'learn the principle' approach

With this idea in mind, even if participants are asked to perform a procedure they should learn the basic principles behind it and how to apply it in different contexts. This approach is partly implemented in screen-based simulators that allow users to practice approaching a specific type of patient (e.g. unconscious for unknown reasons). Also mannikin-based simulations focusing on CRM often follow this approach. The CRM principles (Table 13.2) can serve as prototypical examples for such principles. By conducting scenarios that can be solved better by using those principles, experiences are created in which the principles were helpful. During the following debriefing, participants and instructors discuss where the principles could be helpful and what they mean for medical practice. This approach requires a high plausibility and relevance of the simulated cases. Only if participants accept the scenario as relevant for their practice will they accept such principles as useful.

The 'anticipation-centred' approach

A third learning mode can be called the *anticipation-centred approach* and is also somewhat related to focusing on principles.[42] However, it is less about directly transferring what was learned during the simulation, be it specific skills or general principles. This approach focuses on helping participants to see their clinical reality in new ways. The goal is to help participants improve their professional anticipations in the clinical setting. Anticipations guide actions by helping humans to set goals and by predicting the future development of the situation in which they are acting; as such they are highly relevant when diagnosing and treating a patient. Simulation-based training can serve to widen and deepen anticipation. Widening means that more aspects of a situation can be projected into the future and deepening means projecting further into the future. For example, consider a young participant in a CRM-related course who tries a position as leader in the operating theatre during a vital crisis of the patient. The scenario can be constructed in a way to show potential difficulties whilst doing so (e.g. reversing existing hierarchies, dealing with resistances and own doubts). The participants could then discuss and reflect such different aspects during debriefing. Should a similar (or even different) situation arise in clinical practice this person might have a better picture of what to expect from the situation and could act with improved anticipations.

In the current simulator practice all three approaches are often mixed and less clear cut. In the future it will be necessary to find more and better ways to conduct scenarios in an even more goal-oriented fashion than it is done today. Currently taking part in simulator-courses is not a regular part of continuous medical education in most countries. Optimising the use of simulators and simulations will mean advancing simulation from being a one-time eye-opening event to a systematic part of the medical curriculum. In this regard, simulation in medicine needs to catch up with the aviation industry, which acknowledges the fact that, especially in teaching CRM, there is a need for initial indoctrination, recurrent training, and continuous reinforcement.[43] Medicine is still struggling with the first step.

Different forms of simulators

The different targets for learning require different methods and are applicable to different contents. It is important to match the right educational tool, and especially the way in which it is used, to the right target. An overview of different simulation tools and application areas can be found in the work of Rall and Gaba.[6]

Recently a new type of simulator has become available: baby-sized simulation manikins that simulate a child of about 3 months old. This new development closes an important gap in training opportunities.[44,45,46] On the one hand with medical advances, reduced birth rates, etc. there is less opportunity to become involved in the treatment of newborn babies, and few healthcare professionals actually gain experience with such patients. Whilst on the other hand, in the pre-hospital environment, for example, many healthcare professionals come into contact with emergencies involving newborn babies. Consequently, baby simulators have a high potential for increasing patient safety by allowing for gaining experiences.

Model-based or script-based

We want to focus on one more feature of patient simulators that is discussed increasingly: namely the advantages and disadvantages of model-based vs. script-based simulators. It is often stated that model-based simulators are best, because they are more realistic. With script-based or even manually controlled simulators it might happen more often that slight physiological inconsistencies occur – although there are no studies on this topic. However, one might question the purpose of striving for realism. Especially for educational purposes it might be beneficial or even necessary to deviate from realism to improve learning. We already mentioned some physiological 'helps' that instructors frequently provide to simulation participants to help them learn. Such moves are not easy in model-based simulators, which provide less direct ways to control the simulated physiological processes. Trying to keep the patient alive during a simulation scenario often adds much complexity with model-based simulators. We think it is important to emphasise the learning, not the realism, which might possibly be achieved more easily using script-based simulators that allow for more control of the scenario.

Challenges for simulator instructors

Using simulators for educational purposes poses some challenges for simulator instructors. The tools and their control are complex. The (patho-) physiology of the simulated patient must be simulated, as well as the patient in a more or less interactive role play. Scenarios must be designed and conducted according to the goals, integrating role-playing persons (participants and simulator team), using medical equipment, and also controlling audio/video recording devices. During a running simulator-based course the instructors do take on different roles. In the beginning they mostly instruct how to use the simulator, familiarising the participants with the simulator and the simulated infrastructure. They might also give presentations on theoretical backgrounds of the topics of the course (e.g. crisis resource management, principles of difficult airway management, etc.). During the scenario instructors are 'directors', trying to enable participants to create relevant experiences. During the debriefings that follow, instructors might become facilitators who help participants to learn by themselves. Simulation is a powerful agent that has many desired effects but can also have undesired effects on participants if not used with care. For this complex task, simulator instructors do need some training.

Meanwhile, there are some institutions that offer training courses for healthcare professionals who want to use simulators for training: e.g. Stanford and Boston (USA), Copenhagen (Denmark) and London (England), to name but a few. We have developed the Instructor and Facilitation Training (InFacT)[31,47] and co-operate with the simulation centres in Copenhagen and London in running a European Simulator Instructor Course.[48,49]

Non-educational uses of simulators

In terms of research there are many projects that try to improve the understanding of why simulators and simulations work in reaching their goal. Studies investigate, for example, the effectiveness of simulator training,[50,51,52] and also factors that are important when designing simulator settings on a more process-oriented level.[15,53,54,55] Furthermore, simulators and simulations are increasingly used to undertake research on various human factor topics[56] such as fatigue,[57,58,59] team work[60] and failures of prospective memory[61] as well as ergonomic design and testing of medical devices.[62,63,64]

Using simulators and simulations for assessment is still under much debate.[65,66,67,68,69,70,71,72,73] From a psychometric perspective the main advantage of using simulators and simulations for performance assessment is the (theoretical) reproducibility and objectivity of simulation scenarios. Additional tools are needed to actually record and score participants' performance during scenarios. There are both medical/technical scores[68,69,74,75,76,77,78] and non-technical scores,[79,80,81,82] which in themselves provide higher or lower psychometric quality in terms of validity and reliability. Such assessments can also be used in a formative sense to discover potentials for improvements in participants.

Future developments

We have already touched upon the need to further investigate the processes that make simulation successful. Another major step forward in using simulation in anaesthesiology is to link simulation to incident reporting and analysis.[83,84,85,86] Incident reporting systems (IRS) have developed rapidly worldwide, especially in anaesthesia. The idea is to provide a platform in which healthcare professionals can anonymously report problems (and also good solutions) from clinical practice. Incident reporting systems shift the focus away from individual failure to system issues and error-prone situations within the system. Incident reporting systems are very relevant as they allow for open discussion of problems, protected by anonymity.

There are two ways in which IRS might be connected to simulation. Firstly reported cases in IRS are used to design relevant scenarios for simulation. Incident reporting systems show the bandwidth of what actually happens in clinical practice and thus allow for a closer look behind what *should* be happening. The second way of combining simulation and IRS takes the opposite direction. Some case reports are not very clear and it is hard to understand how the reported problem could evolve. Using an approach called *synthesising error analysis*,[87] it is possible to use simulation to get an improved understanding of a single case in an IRS: the idea is to replicate the case in simulation and to systematically change its context to see under which conditions the problem would evolve or not evolve.[88] Using this approach, for example, it would be possible to better understand the circumstances under which medication errors, like dosage errors or mix-ups, might happen.

In order to find countermeasures, a deeper understanding of error-prone situations, root causes and moderating factors is needed. Overall understanding when and why humans make errors is not clear enough. To use a metaphor: if a patient arrives in a hospital it would not be enough to say that she or he is ill. To treat this person, more details are needed. The same holds for addressing human error.

A final conceptual addition to current simulator training is *prospective simulation*[89] combining the ideas of failure modes and effect analysis (FMEA) with simulation. The basic idea of FMEA is to cognitively simulate certain processes, e.g. a difficult intubation, and to think through what could go wrong during this process (e.g. certain equipment might not be available). Simulators allow constant modification to such processes, making it possible to create more threats and thus to question habitual approaches, find better solutions and more effective countermeasures. Simulating the process with actual equipment, combined with the ability to stop processes, rewind, change, and reflect upon approaches can help to widen and deepen anticipation. This approach is especially fruitful with '*in situ*' simulation and video-assisted debriefings as it allows discussion very close to actual practice.

Summary

Simulation and simulators in their various forms have the potential to increase patient safety. Further conceptual and technological developments of simulation will advance the current educational use of simulators from one-time appetisers to real, systematic and recurrent training. Simulation needs to be integrated not only in an educational curriculum, but also in health care organisations and the medical field. Anaesthesia has a leading role in this regard but there are also some more steps to take.

Simulation can become a catalyst in building a safety culture and can become an important element of systematic improvements of patient safety as a system. Throughout the process of becoming or being an anaesthesiologist, simulation can help in reducing potential threats to patient safety, both in number and severity. The number of first attempts with patients can be reduced when simulation is used systematically where appropriate. The first contacts of medical students with patients can in many regards be better prepared using simulation. For healthcare professionals simulation can also become an even more powerful tool for learning new skills, procedures, principles, and for widening and deepening their anticipation, especially with regard to the very important crisis resource management. There is a lot of face validity, albeit if only little data showing that simulation does help to increase competencies. After a simulation-based CRM course participants use terminology to concisely describe phenomena in treating patients for which they did not have the words before, even if they knew the phenomenon as such. Understanding those concepts and accepting them as an integrated part of medical professionalism helps in addressing and ultimately reducing human (and system) error. Open discussions and constructive feedback in the safe simulator environment about strengths and weaknesses in participants' approaches to cases might establish the groundwork for a safety culture in which everybody tries to optimise patient safety and not find a bad apple who committed a mistake.

References

1. Cooper JB, Gaba D. No myth: anesthesia is a model for addressing patient safety. *Anesthesiology* 2002; **97**: 1335–7.
2. Gaba DM. Anaesthesiology as a model for patient safety in health care. *BMJ* 2000; **320**: 785–8.
3. Henson LC, Lee AC, eds. *Simulators in Anesthesiology Education*. New York: Plenum Press, 1998.
4. Gaba DM. A brief history of mannequin-based simulation application. In Dunn WF, ed. *Simulators in Critical Care and Beyond*. Des Plaines, IL: Society of Critical Care Medicine, 2004, pp. 7–14.
5. Dunn WF, ed. *Simulators in Critical Care and Beyond*. Des Plaines, IL: Society of Critical Care Medicine, 2004.
6. Rall M, Gaba DM. Patient simulators. In Miller RD, ed. *Anaesthesia*. New York: Elsevier, 2005, pp. 3073–103.
7. Gaba DM. The future vision of simulation in health care. *Qual Saf Health Care* 2004; **13** (Suppl 1): i2–10.
8. Rall M, Stricker E, Reddersen S, Zieger J, Dieckmann P. Mobile 'in-situ' crisis resource management training: simulator courses with video-assisted debriefing where participants work. In Kyle R, Murray BW, eds., *Clinical Simulation: Operations, Engineering, and Management* 2007.
9. Dieckmann P, Rall M. Becoming a simulator instructor and learning to facilitate: the Instructor and Facilitation Training (InFacT). In Kyle R, Murray BW, eds. *Clinical Simulation: Operations, Engineering, and Management*. Burlington, MA: Elsevier, 2007.
10. Kneebone RL, Kidd J, Nestel D, *et al*. Blurring the boundaries: scenario-based simulation in a clinical setting. *Med Educ* 2005; **39**: 580–7.
11. Komich N. CRM Scenario development: the next generation. In Jensen RS, ed. *Proceedings of the Sixth International Symposium on Aviation Psychology*. Vol I. Columbus, OH: Ohio State University, 1991, pp. 53–9.
12. Murray BW. Simulators in critical care education: educational aspects & building scenarios. In Dunn WF, ed. *Simulators in Critical Care and Beyond*. Des Plaines, IL: Society of Critical Care Medicine, 2004, pp. 29–32.
13. Prince C, Oser R, Salas E, Woodruff W. Increasing hits and reducing misses in CRM/LOS scenarios: guidlines for simulator scenario development. *The International Journal of Aviation Psychology* 1993; **3**: 69–82.
14. Dieckmann P. *"Ein bisschen wirkliche Echtheit simulieren": Über Simulatorsettings in der Anästhesiologie ("Simulating a Little Bit of True Reality": On Simulator Settings in Anaesthesiology)*. Doctoral Dissertation, Carl-von-Ossietzky University Oldenburg, 2005. Oldenburg: Universität, Dissertation, 2005.

15. Dieckmann P, Manser T, Wehner T, Rall M. Reality and fiction cues in medical patient simulation. An interview study with anesthesiologists. *Journal of Cognitive Engineering and Decision Making*, in press.

16. Gaba DM. Human error in anesthetic mishaps. *Int Anesthesiol Clin* 1989; **27**: 137–47.

17. Gaba DM. Dynamic decision making in anesthesiology: cognitive models and training approaches. In Evans DA, Patel VL, eds. *Advanced Models of Cognition for Medical Training and Practice*. Berlin: Springer, 1992; pp. 123–47.

18. Gaba DM, DeAnda A. A comprehensive anesthesia simulation environment: re-creating the operating room for research and training. *Anesthesiology* 1988; **69**: 387–94.

19. Gaba DM, Fish K J, Howard SK. *Crisis Management in Anesthesiology*. Philadelphia, MA: Churchill Livingstone, 1994.

20. Howard SK, Gaba D, Fish KJ, Yang GCB, Sarnquist FH. Anesthesia crisis resource management training: teaching anesthesiologists to handle critical incidents. *Aviat Space Environ Med* 1992; **63**: 763–70.

21. Cooper JB, Newborner RS, Kitz RJ. An analysis of major errors and equipment failures in anesthesia management: considerations for prevention and detection. *Anesthesiology* 1984; **60**: 34–42.

22. Cooper JB, Newborner RS, Long CD, Philip JH. Preventable anesthesia mishaps: a study of human factors. *Anesthesiology* 1978; **49**: 399–406.

23. Runciman WB, Webb RK, Lee R, Holland R. The Australian Incident Monitoring Study. System failure: an analysis of 2000 incident reports. *Anaesth Intensive Care* 1993; **21**: 684–95.

24. Barach P, Berwick DM. Patient safety and the reliability of health care systems. *Ann Intern Med* 2003; **138**: 997–8.

25. Rall M, Gaba DM. Human Performance and Patient Safety. In Miller RD, ed. *Miller's Anaesthesia*. Philadelphia, MA: Elsevier Churchill Livingston, 2005; pp. 3021–72.

26. Rall M, Manser T, Guggenberger H, Gaba DM, Unertl K. Patientensicherheit und Fehler in der Medizin. Entstehung, Prävention und Analyse von Zwischenfällen. *Anästhesiol Intensivmed Notfallmed Schmerzther* 2001; **36**: 321–30.

27. Kohn LT, Corrigan JM, Donaldson MS, eds. *To Err is Human. Building a Safer Health System*, http://www.nap.edu/books/0309068371/html/. Washington, DC: National Academy of Science, 2000.

28. Committee on Quality of Health Care in America. *Crossing the Quality Chiasm: A New Health System for the 21st Century*. Washington, DC: National Academy Press, 2001.

29. Rall M, Dieckmann P. Simulation and patient safety. The use of simulation to enhance patient safety on a system level. *Curr Anaesth Crit Care* 2005; **16**: 273–81.

30. van Meurs W, Mönk S. *Proposed Terminology for Educational Acute Care Simulators*. Abstracts of the Annual Meeting of the Society on Europe for Simulation Applied to Medicine (SESAM), Stockholm, Sweden, June 2004, www.sesam2004.se/complete_abstracts.pdf; Aufgerufen am 13. Juli 2004, 2004.

31. Dieckmann P, Rall M. Designing a scenario as a simulated clinical experience: the TuPASS scenario script. In Kyle R, Murray BW, eds. *Clinical Simulation: Operations, Engineering, and Management*, 2007.

32. Hays RT, Singer MJ. *Simulation Fidelity in Training System Design: Bridging the Gap Between Reality and Training.* New York: Springer, 1989.
33. Feinstein AH, Cannon HM. Constructs of simulation evaluation. *Simulation and Gaming* 2002; **33**: 425–40.
34. Mann JH. Experimental evaluations of role playing. *Psychol Bull* 1956; **53**: 227–34.
35. Schaedle B, Dieckmann P, Wengert A, Zieger J, Rall M. The role of debriefing in simulator training courses for medical students (Abstract Santander-02–20). *European Journal of Anaesthesiology* 2003; **20**: 850.
36. Reason J. *Human Error.* Cambridge: Cambridge University Press, 1990.
37. Dieckmann P, Reddersen S, Zieger J, Rall M. A structure for video-assisted debriefing in simulator-based training of crisis resource management. In Kyle R, Murray BW, eds. *Clinical Simulation: Operations, Engineering, and Management.* Burlington, MA: Elsevier, 2007.
38. Dieckmann P, Rall M. Becoming a simulator instructor and learning to facilitate: the instructor and facilitation training (InFacT). In Kyle R, Murray BW, eds. *Clinical Simulation: Operations, Engineering, and Management.* Burlington, MA: Elsevier, 2007.
39. Timmermann A, Eich C, Nickel E, Russo S, *et al.* Simulation and airway management. *Anaesthesist* 2005; **54**: 582–7.
40. Rall M, Stricker E, Reddersen S, Dieckmann P. *Train Where you Work. Mobile 'In-situ' Simulation Training with Video-assisted Debriefing in Different Acute Care Settings,* http://www.euroanesthesia.org/education/refreshcourses.php. ESA Refresher Course 2005.
41. Leontjew AA. *Activity, Consciousness, Personality.* Englewood Cliffs, NJ: Prentice-Hall, 1978.
42. Stadler M, Wehner T. Anticipation as a basic principle in goal-directed action. In Freese M, Sabini J, eds. *Goal-directed Behavior: The Concept of Action in Psychology.* Hillsdale, NJ: Lawrence Erlbaum Associates inc., 1985, pp. 67–77.
43. Federal Aviation Administration. *Crew Resource Management Training.* Advisory Circular No. 120-51D, 2001.
44. Blike GT, Christoffersen K, Cravero JP, Andeweg SK, Jensen J. A method for measuring system safety and latent errors associated with pediatric procedural sedation. *Anesth Analg* 2005; **101**: 48–58.
45. Weinstock PH, Kappus LJ, Kleinman ME, *et al.* Toward a new paradigm in hospital-based pediatric education: the development of an onsite simulator program. *Pediatr Crit Care Med* 2005; **6**: 635–41.
46. Eich C, Russo S, Timmermann A, Nickel EA, Graf BM. New perspectives for simulator-based training in paediatric anaesthesia and emergency medicine. *Anaesthesist* 2006; **55**: 179–84.
47. Dieckmann P, Rall M. Becoming a simulator instructor and learning to facilitate: the Instructor and Facilitation Training – InFacT. *Simulation in Health Care* 2006; **1**: 103.
48. Östergaard D, Dieckmann P, Rall M, *et al. Train the Trainers Programme for Full-Scale Simulation Facilitators.* Poster presented at the AMEE Meeting, Genoa, 2006.
49. Dieckmann P, Rall M, Östergaard H, *et al. European Instructor Course for Simulator Instructors: Concept and Evaluation Data.* Presentation at the SESAM Meeting, Bristol, 2005.

50. Østergard D, Jensen PF, Jacobson J, *et al*. Does training in a full-scale anesthesia simulator improve residents' performance? *Anesthesiology* 1997; **87**: A940.

51. Abrahamson S, Denson JS, Wolf RM. Effectiveness of a simulator in training anesthesiology residents. *J Med Educ* 1969; **44**: 515–19.

52. Tan GM, Ti LK, Suresh S, Ho BS, Lee TL. Teaching first-year medical students physiology: does the human patient simulator allow for more effective teaching? *Singapore Med J* 2002; **43**: 238–42.

53. Salas E, Burke CS. Simulation for training is effective when . . . *Qual Saf Health Care* 2002; **11**: 119–20.

54. Issenberg SB, McGaghie WC, Petrusa ER, Lee Gordon D, Scalese RJ. Features and uses of high-fidelity medical simulations that lead to effective learning: a BEME systematic review. *Med Teach* 2005; **27**: 10–28.

55. Manser T, Dieckmann P, Wehner T, Rall M. Comparison of anaesthetists' activity patterns in the operating room and during simulation. *Ergonomics* 2007; **50**: 246–60.

56. Gaba DM. Research techniques in human performance using realistic simulation. In Henson LC, Lee AC, eds. *Simulators in Anesthesiology Education*. New York: Plenum Press, 1998, pp. 93–102.

57. Howard SK, Smith BE, Daba DM, Rosekind MR. Performance of well-rested vs. highly-fatigued residents: a simulator study. *Anesthesiology* 1997; **87**: A981.

58. Gaba DM, Howard SK. Fatigue among clinicians and the safety of patients. *N Engl J Med* 2002; **347**: 1249–55.

59. Howard SK, Keshavacharya S, Smith BE, *et al*. Behavioral evidence of fatigue during a simulator experiment. *Anesthesiology* 1998; **89**: A1236.

60. Manser T, Howard SK, Gaba D. *An Observation Method to Assess Coordination Processes in Anesthesia*, http://www.anestech.org/media/Publications/IMMS_2005/Manser.pdf. 2005.

61. Dieckmann P, Reddersen S, Wehner T, Rall M. Prospective memory failures as an unexplored threat to patient safety: results from a pilot study using patient simulators to investigate the missed execution of intentions. *Ergonomics* 2006; **49**: 526–43.

62. Agutter J, Drews F, Syroid N, *et al*. Evaluation of graphic cardiovascular display in a high-fidelity simulator. *Anesth Analg* 2003; **97**: 1403–13.

63. Gurushanthaiah K, Weinger MB, Englund CE. Visual display format affects the ability of anesthesiologists to detect acute physiologic changes. A laboratory study employing a clinical display simulator. *Anesthesiology* 1995; **83**: 1184–93.

64. Syroid ND, Agutter J, Drews FA, *et al*. Development and evaluation of a graphical anesthesia drug display. *Anesthesiology* 2002; **96**: 565–75.

65. Bond WF, Spillane L. The use of simulation for emergency medicine resident assessment. *Acad Emerg Med* 2002; **9**: 1295–9.

66. Devitt JH, Kurrek MM, Cohen MM, Cleave-Hogg D. The validity of performance assessments using simulation. *Anesthesiology* 2001; **95**: 36–42.

67. Gaba DM, Botney R, Howard SK, Fish KJ, Flanagan B. Interrater-reliability of performance assessment tools for the management of simulated anesthetic crisis. *Anesthesiology* 1994; **81**: A1277.

68. Gaba DM, Howard SK, Flanagan B, *et al*. Assessment of clinical performance during simulated crises using both technical and behavioral ratings. *Anesthesiology* 1998; **89**: 8–18.

69. Issenberg SB, McGaghie WC, Hart IR, *et al*. Simulation technology for health care professional skills training and assessment. *JAMA* 1999; **282**: 861–6.

70. Weller JM, Bloch M, Young S, *et al*. Evaluation of high-fidelity patient simulator in assessment of performance of anaesthetists. *Br J Anaesth* 2003; **90**: 43–7.

71. Forrest F, Taylor MA, Postlethwaite K, Aspinall R. Use of a high-fidelity simulator to develop testing of the technical performance of novice anaesthetists. *Br J Anaesth* 2002; **88**: 228–344.

72. Gaba DM, Small SD. How can full environment-realistic patient simulators be used for performance assessment. *Newsletter of the American Society of Anesthesiologists* 1997; **61**: 9–12.

73. Morgan PJ, Cleave-Hogg D, Guest CB, Herold J. Validity and reliability of undergraduate performance assessments in an anesthesia simulator. *Can J Anesthesiol* 2001; **48**: 225–33.

74. Harrison TK, Manser T, Howard SK, Gaba DM. Use of cognitive AIDS in a simulated anesthetic crisis. *Anesth Analg* 2006; **103**: 551–6.

75. Byrne AJ, Greaves JD. Assessment instruments used during anaesthetic simulation: review of published studies. *Br J Anaesth* 2001; **86**: 445–50.

76. Glavin RJ, Maran NJ. Development and use of scoring systems for assessment of clinical competence. *Br J Anaesth* 2002; **88**: 329–30.

77. Goodwin MW, French GW. Simulation as a training and assessment tool in the management of failed intubation in obstetrics. *Int J Obstet Anesth* 2001; **10**: 273–7.

78. Tome JA, Fletcher J, Lydell DR. Performance assessment of medical students educated in a simulator environment. *Anesthesiology* 1997; **87**: A944.

79. Gaba DM, Lee T. Measuring the workload of the anesthesiologist. *Anesth Analg* 1990; **71**: 354–61.

80. Weinger MB, Herndon OW, Zornow MH, *et al*. An objective methodology for task analysis and workload assessment in anesthesia providers. *Anesthesiology* 1994; **80**: 77–92.

81. Fletcher G, Flin R, McGeorge P, *et al*. Anaesthetists' Non-Technical Skills (ANTS): evaluation of a behavioural marker system. *Br J Anaesth* 2003; **90**: 580–8.

82. Fletcher GCL, McGeorge P, Flin RH, Glavin RJ, Maran NJ. The role of non-technical skills in anaesthesia: a review of current literature. *Br J Anaesth* 2002; **88**: 419–29.

83. Leape L. Reporting of adverse events. *N Engl J Med* 2002; **347**: 1633–8.

84. Rall M, Martin J, Geldner G, *et al*. Charakteristika effektiver Incident-Reporting-Systeme zur Erhöhung der Patientensicherheit. *Anästhesiol Intensivmed Notfallmed* 2006: S9–19.

85. Stanhope N, Crowley-Murphy M, Vincent C, O'Connor AM, Taylor-Adams SE. An evaluation of adverse incident reporting. *Journal of Evaluation in Clinical Practice* 1999; **5**: 5–12.

86. Vincent CA. Analysis of clinical incidents: a window on the system, not a search for root causes. *Qual Saf Health Care* 2004; **13**: 242–3.

87. Mehl K, Schuette M. Simulators: a perspective on what to train and what to analyse regarding human reliability. In Scheller GI, Kaffka P, eds. *Safety and Reliability*. Rotterdam, Brookfiel: A. A. Balkema, 1999, pp. 675–680.

88. Dieckmann P, Rall M, Östergaard D. The role of patient simulation and incident reporting in the development and evaluation of medical devices and the training of their users. *Work*, accepted.

89. Dieckmann P, Wehner T, Rall M, Manser T. Prospektive simulation: Ein Konzept zur methodischen Ergänzung von medizinischen Simulatorsettings. *Zeitschrift für Arbeitswissenschaft* 2005; **59**: 172–80.

Index

Note: page numbers in *italics* refer to figures and tables.